To Anne Dean
fellow inquirer
with appreciation and
best wishes —
Bill Respdz

TRAUMA ENERGETICS

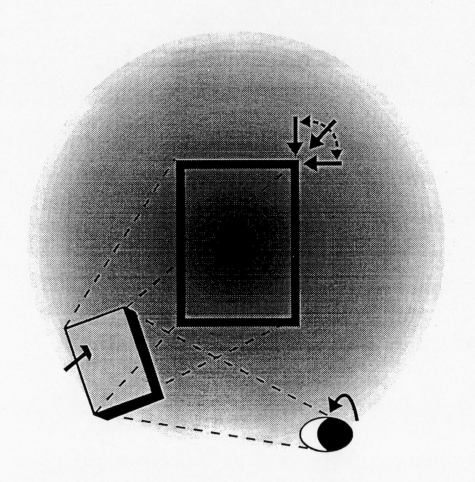

Patterns

TRAUMA ENERGETICS

A Study of Held-Energy Systems

William M. Redpath

Barberry Press

LEXINGTON, MASSACHUSETTS
1995

Trauma Energetics, Held-Energy Systems SM, a process for educating individuals about how trauma is stored in the mindbody, is patent pending.
Trauma Energetics, Held-Energy Systems SM, is a trade/service mark with registration applied for.

Grateful acknowledgement is made for the use of the following copyrighted material: Excerpt from "Oedipus at Colonus" in SOPHOCLES: THE OEDIPUS CYCLE: AN ENGLISH VERSION by Dudley Fitts and Robert Fitzgerald.(pp.162-163), copyright 1949 by Harcourt Brace & Company and renewed 1977 by Cornelia Fitts and Robert Fitzgerald, reprinted by permission of the publisher. CAUTION: All rights, including professional, amateur, motion picture, recitation, lecturing, public reading, radio broadcasting, and television are strictly reserved. Inquiries on all rights should be addressed to Harcourt Brace & Company, Permission Department, Orlando, Florida.32887-6777.

Library of Congress Catalogue Card Number 95-94856

Redpath, William M., 1940-
      Trauma Energetics, A Study of Held-Energy Systems / William M. Redpath
      ISBN 0-9467730-0-7
      1.Self-Healing 2. Mind and Body. 3. Education 4. Trauma

For information address: Barberry Press, 02173-8025. 617-861-0184

Printed in **Lexington, Massachusetts**
First Edition, Version 1.0
First Printing

For my mother, For Judy,

and in memory of my father

CONTENTS

ACKNOWLEDGEMENTS   ix

INTRODUCTION: A JOURNEY BEGINS   1

CHAPTER ONE: MORE JOURNEY   25

CHAPTER TWO: TRAUMA AND HELD ENERGY   57

CHAPTER THREE: ON BLACK   97

CHAPTER FOUR: TECHNIQUE CONSIDERATIONS   131

CHAPTER FIVE: FURTHER STRATEGIES AND
     ANECDOTES   153

CHAPTER SIX: A SESSION   165

CHAPTER SEVEN: ENERGY, THE SPIRIT, AND
     RELIGION   291

CHAPTER EIGHT: CHRISTIANS AND JEWS   315

CHAPTER NINE: CHRIST ENERGY AND AUTHORITY   329

APPENDIX: THERAPISTS AND ABUSE   339

GLOSSARY   357

IDIOSYNCRATIC BIBLIOGRAPHY   361

INDEX   365

ACKNOWLEDGEMENTS

I thank my family, friends, and colleagues for their support of me in my process and in friendship, as well as in particular with some, the development of my work and of this technique. I am deeply grateful to you for your responses, suggestions, and insights. I know that what I have set down in total here expresses for the most part, for some of you, not your ideas or opinions at all, though you have contributed to my understanding.

In other words, you bear no responsibility for these ideas and strategies, nor, come to think of it, at some ultimate level, do I. Upon reflection, opinions become increasingly difficult to render. Some of you friends mentioned below do not even know about the text; others have been qualified in their responses and their understanding of what I have attempted here, an exploration of a perspective.

That said, I prize my relationships with you. They are blessings in my life, and I wish to acknowledge them here, particularly the following, including those of you who have helped directly with the evolution of my understanding resulting in this book: Nancy S.M. Redpath, Samuel Fisk, Randall Paulsen, Mark Hochwender, Betsy Gillis, Leslie Sprouse, Caroline Schastny, J.P. Streit, Jr., Carl Brauer, Myron Sharaf, Stephanie Mines, Anna Hyder, Connie Boyer, Wilhelm Heppe, Kenneth McElheny, Timothy Sens, Charles Dietrick, Michael Ponsor, Joseph Pleck, Richard Paul, Frances Mervyn, Haskell Cohen, Robert Yuhnke, Nancy Schieffelin, Richard Stendstadtvold, Susan Melchior, Priscilla Mueller, John Latz, Christian Muller, Charles Fisk, Virginia Frecha, Linda Coe, Sally Bowie, George and Hilary Newman, Matthew Newman, my brave and trusting clients, my brother Robert, my sisters Nancy and Jean, and in growth and connection, my wife, Judith Jordan.

I have received so much from my teachers, including Vimala Thakar, Stacey Mills, again Myron Sharaf, Emmet Hutchins, Peter Melchior, Peter Levine, Tom Wing, Henry LaFleur, Rosemary Keene, George Dillenger, Gregge Tiffen, John Pierrakos, Stephen Fleck, Thomas Henn, Alois Nagler, and Alan Wilkinson. I thank you all for your teachings and for the opportunities to learn.

Gratitude also to my thoughtful readers, who slogged through this text, offering creative suggestions and commentary, including Nancy S.M. Redpath, Mark Hochwender, Myron Sharaf, Samuel Fisk, Kenneth McElheny, Jean Garrison, Florence Trefethen, J.P. Streit, Jr., and Carolyn Schastny.

I also wish to thank Marilyn Claff particularly, Mary Curran, and Charles McKenna for their skill and support in getting this book into publishable, published form. Also my appreciation to Margot Geffen for her graphics expertise in executing the cover and frontispiece.

Please note that the descriptions of client history are composites and are disguised to protect client privacy. It is interesting to note that for purposes of the perspective I am rendering, the descriptions of sessions contain little that could be considered confidential, in the narrative sense of the word.

INTRODUCTION: A JOURNEY BEGINS

Orientation

In the tradition of Friends (Quakers) and of Vimala Thakar, this book is addressed to friends—fellow inquirers into the nature of awareness—and as such has a somewhat personal, varied structure. I begin with a description of my own process as a way of conveying how I achieved the point of view I am presenting. A discussion of trauma and a method I have found to unlock traumatic patterning follows, as does the transcript of a complete session using the technique with a client. I conclude with chapters applying this perspective to themes in religion, spirituality, and therapist abuse.

Not every part of this book will seem relevant to all friends, known and unknown. You are welcome to browse, share, overlook, and play. Eventually, I hope a holistic continuity of perspective will emerge between the various parts. Also I hope you will come to understand that this book is about energetic experience, not ideas or words, which describe it.

In response to readers' suggestions, I want to say that I am not trying to persuade the unpersuadable, nor to prove scientifically anything in what follows. To interface between language and energy appears to be regularly problematic. What follows is inquiry, an invitation to share the experiences initiating or surrounding these insights. These energetics are the places of first and last resort. Even words, or the ideas they express can be seen to be beside the point.

+ + +

Friends:

I am seven years old, in my own back yard in suburban New Jersey, chasing my older sister as fast as I can run. She takes an unusual path through my family's rotting picnic-table platform behind the garage, and suddenly, below me, I see the gleaming, thick fragment of an old Becker's Dairy milk bottle amid the weeds, and know my body is heading for it. Instantly set into slow, eternal motion, I try to twist away, but my momentum carries me floating, unable to prevent the arch of my foot from crashing with full force upon the upright edge of embedded glass.

Sitting calmly in a chair some forty-six years later in Boulder, Colorado, in a partial way I reexperience total body agony as my left arch is deeply penetrated by the thick, sharp shard. I sense again the slow motion of my fall, the altered perception of time in my head and body, somehow uniquely free. Then dragging myself back toward the house. I hear again my own cries break the Sunday afternoon calm.

After this cut, I know something has shifted radically. Some childhood sense of invulnerability and perfection has been challenged by the information the glass sends blasting through my brain. And I have a pre-impact vision of time and space I have never consciously experienced before.

You know how in the first flush of considering a new idea, every aspect of life can become interrelated to that idea as over time our brain integrates the new levels of information contained in or surrounding the insight. In 1993, in Boulder, after taking a short workshop with Peter Levine, a noted teacher and expert on trauma, and after a trauma *renegotiation* session (his technique) with him, I found myself turning yet another corner in my understanding of the nature of trauma, a phenomenon I had been examining both academically and with clients for over three decades.

In my session with Peter, I choose to work on this childhood incident, and he and I reassemble the scattered segments of my memory: How slowly the adults seem to respond, how a kitchen roller hand towel hesitantly is placed around my rapidly bleeding foot—is the towel going to be ruined?

Someone offers me reassurance, but I am too anxious, and they seem concerned as well. Someone calls our doctor—not available. I get into the back seat of our family car, with its curved fenders. A bathtowel now protects the cushion from my blood, and my father drives me to the office of another doctor I have met once or twice before at a family party.

I remember my dread. My foot needs stitches. The doctor says there is no need for anaesthetic, because it won't take that long. My father is uncharacteristically aloof and silent with me. Is he angry to have his nap so disturbed? He holds my leg down upon the examining table. I am in anticipatory panic, and I shout as the doctor stitches up my foot.

In a second phase, I scream louder, expressing a deeper sense of rage at not feeling cared for—perhaps the situation had started with some sibling quarrel, or there had been trouble earlier in the weekend which led me to such feeling, not one I was used to acknowledging. At one point, the doctor suggests that I do not need to yell so hard; he does not believe it hurts that much.

Peter has me explore the situation, at one point advising me to focus upon the scene and its colors as a way of vivifying and diluting (he calls it *titrating*) the toxicity of the memory.

"I can see the green-red tomatoes on the high shelf of the screened-in back porch," I report.

"Focus upon the wires of the screen," he suggests. I feel a shift as I enter the black of the screen weave. "Head for the black of the screen; that is where the energy is held," Peter offers.

At the time, I do not quite understand what he means. Is the memory a form of traumatically fixed energy? Or, as I sensed and was later to view it, is the black itself *life energy* traumatically immobilized? In physics, black means absence of movement. For some moments in the chair, I now sense that with color, I can again "enter" what I had come to think of as *the energetic*, as I once did with John Pierrakos, a neo-Reichian bioenergetic practitioner and theoretician.

Pierrakos and My Body's Aura

In the 1970s, Pierrakos had encouraged me not to dismiss the radiant haze which I saw around my fingers, but rather to consider it as a way to envision my body's otherwise invisible aura with another sight, acknowledging its "palpable," literal, vibrational reality. By focusing upon the sensation, here color, I could hover apperceptively between particle and wave understanding. What I sensed was somehow true. To that experience was now being added another in my growing assembly of encounters with energy in my mindbody.

As I progressed more deeply into the memory of my foot trauma, I intuited from the evidence of my current sensations recollected in tranquilly in Peter's office, that the doctor was not keeping the anaesthetic from me for the reason he said. With some deep movement, I sensed there had been no anaesthetic available, and the doctor did not want to frighten me further with the absolute irremediability of the pain he was going to inflict, nor of my terror at the prospect of pain and even death.

As I connected with this more complex reality in the renegotiation session, I was moved to tears by the compassion I felt for him and for my father, who now seemed more anxious than aloof. Something deep and fixed about the memory softened, and I felt stress leave my mind and body, as my predominate emotion revealed more concern for them and their reality than for myself; I felt empathy where before I sensed the remembered situation was locked in a blunt, cartoon kind of forgetting.

Over the many months since that session, I have turned the sensations and feelings surrounding this traumatic incident into an avocation, almost like a hobby, progressing incrementally by various means, including significantly the techniques presented in this book, until I have cleared out most of its toxicity. My mindbody does not have to detour around the neurochemistry of the trauma and its stored memory.

At times I have experienced excruciating pain in my left foot and elsewhere as I chased the pattern down to a series of moments wherein the glass enters the skin of my left arch, sending radical sensations throughout my mindbody. Each new layer has a threshold of toxicity which I pass through, into deeper and deeper resolution of the patterns which were so catastrophically set in.

This crisis-memorial has been a demanding and marvelous teacher. For from these experiences, I can report that the effect of this occasion upon the alignment of my body and me within it, in my current estimate, was profound. Something happened after the accident—I lost touch with my center—my groin, my gut, and my solar plexus, my diaphragm. In Japanese terms, I disconnected from my *hara* energy; using another eastern strategy, chakra access throughout the lower half of my body was compromised.

And while I quickly recovered significant sense of my early, happy self, enough to succeed in many ways, I started to put on weight, becoming, among other sometime realities as well as body image distortions, a fat, depressed, uncoordinated boy, with an unconscious limp, a fate which radically transformed my inner sense of myself as whole.

Certainly there were many additional factors determining these shifts. The way I envision trauma now is that single traumata may be catastrophic in impact, carrying a deterministic spin which seems chancy, irrevocable, and unfair. Trauma also proceeds through and describes channels of neurochemistry which are dormant, even awaiting expression and resolution within catastrophe, so that I may not easily attribute all its effects upon one blaming and blamed occasion.

Forty-eight years later, I have only recently reworked the distortions which diets or weight accrual could not effect. Whatever developmental processes put on hold by the trauma now have been reactivated, and at times I move with the enthusiasm and rebalancing energies of a seven year-old. And I continue to hunt for the vestiges of patterning which still contain me.

Whether this trauma occurred exactly as I have recalled and sensed it is not an issue, nor is its centrality in my myth. Most probably, it was emblematic of forces already operant in me, and its

narrative form dovetailed with earlier energetic patterns laid in before
birth. And certainly I went on with my life, the way we all do. What
has become important is the way my mindbody now in slow, small
steps can transform its alignment in response to my ventures into the
pattern it has traumatically stored, even to the sub-cellular level.

My recent recovery and renegotiation of this single trauma has
brought considerable hope and enlightenment to me in the inner place
where before there was no movement. By witnessing this trauma
patterning, I have learned further how trauma is stored and removed,
though in 1993 I realized in fact I had been studying trauma beginning
with my earliest readings and writings about tragedy and tragic theory
while in graduate school in the early 1960s.

Early Studies of Tragedy

My enchantment with the theater was secured by the age of
four, when my parents took me to my first Broadway show, the
original production of *Oklahoma*. My appreciation deepened over
many years, until I found myself studying dramatic literature and
philosophy in England in 1961. I wanted then to understand what my
experience of drama, as spectator, actor, critic, and now writer,
entailed.

Though previously I had enjoyed musicals and comedies, as
well as serious drama, at Cambridge University I was encouraged to
study tragic literature and theories about tragedy, and I felt in some
way I was coming home to a level of committed focus that had been
previously truncated or postponed.

Scanning the history of intellectual endeavor and its
relationship to actual events in recorded and literary history, I kept
stumbling over the lack of connection between ideas and experience
within the following critical fact. No matter how well-intentioned, as
humans we still cripple and destroy ourselves and others, physically
and emotionally.

If we concentrate on objective experience to describe how we
end up in bad places, our repetition of negative patterns seems rarely

circumscribed, and then usually tyrannically. We still promulgate suffering and pain as well as endure them.

I thought there must be another level beyond what I had been studying in the history of thought and feeling which could be addressed if we are to stop our self-destructive, addictive sequences of behavior and response. And this is what as a graduate student I became interested in: How truly to conclude these sequences of revenge against self and other.

As a child, I was exquisitely responsive to people's pain, openly, spontaneously crying when I saw pathos and suffering in daily life. For this problem, I received various strategies from family, community, and from my education, but I had a growing awareness of the discrepancy I experienced between practice and preaching. Thoughts and related strategies people offered did not stop the cruelty or my sense that people were not aware of what they were doing.

As a pre-adolescent, an acquaintance of mine revealed a fear of banana seeds; apparently her family had been concerned about seeds causing diverticulitis. Ritually, she would peel down one end of the banana and with her finger dig into the end of it until she mushed out the seeds she could see. Then, without further ado, she would eat the rest of the banana whole.

Suggesting that the seeds were not dangerous did not alter her exceptional behavior, and we were left trying to show her that bananas had seeds all through their length. But there was no rationality to her repeated pattern, nor could reason change it.

Over time, I came to see her perhaps exaggerated behavior pattern not as an exception, but as a kind of disturbing rule: People dig out some problem as far as they are inclined or prepossessed to, then proceed without consideration to eat the rest of the banana whole.

As cultures and individuals, why don't we follow through? What happens in the moment when we drop one objective and proceed with our lives, ignoring a whole segment we have started? What does it look like to complete something, not just perpetuate a cycle of, say, revenge, as in the stories surrounding the Trojan War, or of the Mafia? Is it because we ourselves are somehow incomplete, or wounded? This sequence of thought and observation ultimately led me to concerns about finding new ways of addressing our idiosyncratic, perhaps wounded, condition and finally of discovering how, as creatures, to heal ourselves.

What is Tragedy?

The fact that there is something we cannot complete, or are vainly trying to complete, is somehow connected to how we cannot keep ourselves from human disaster. Such a reality quickly evokes our concept of tragedy. I discovered that there are many theories about what tragedy is and is not, yet many people start with Aristotle's lecture notes on tragedy in his *Poetics*. Most people have two basic approaches to a tragedy:
1. Tragedy, in the journalistic sense, is used to describe events such as when children are killed by an oncoming train when their school bus stalls at the railroad crossing. Tragedy is something unwanted and difficult involving grievous early truncation of life and possibility. It has to do with what happens to people.
2. A tragedy is a drama or story, which Aristotle terms *muthos*, which demonstrates the fall (*peripeteia*) from some high, successful place of a hero/scapegoat. These dramas have a specific sad and universal focus upon our experience of suffering. Here tragedy focuses upon some inner human process which may or may not be directly caused by something outside the so-called individual.

No matter how we use the term, when we talk about tragedy, we are usually talking about not just its so-called opposite, comedy, but about something that often preoccupies us as more problematic, sober, and more penetrating, because it characterizes our experiences of suffering and its avoidability. Tragic heroes portray something about the nature and necessity of suffering.

Tragic insight shows how the illusion of unavoidable suffering places us in a disastrous predicament. No matter what we do, we will be inflicted with a disturbance that involves perceived discontinuity and devastation of some, perhaps all aspects of what we think of as ourselves.

In the history of thought, the latter examples from drama have a quasi-technical focus concerning, among other matters, to whom does tragedy occur? Even Aristotle's *Poetics* may be read to show that this is not so easy a question as it first appears. Centuries of exegesis of his notes have yielded only superficial results, when it comes to stopping suffering. If tragedy happens to a hero, what constitutes a hero? Can a society be a hero? Can a woman? Can only a royal person be a hero? What state does he/she fall from and into? What are the roles of fate, determinism, social context, relationship to gods, pride, causality, and similar concerns?

Over the centuries, tragic playwrights as well as theoreticians generally have reflected the understanding of their times. Under the influence of Freud, some recent scholars have interpreted the dramatic tragedies we know, particularly of the ancient Greeks, as re-visits to the realm of trauma: A colossal impact forces us into some kind of serious detour from our usual experience of self.

Of course, tragedies written for the theater describe situations most of us would find stunning and radically, even permanently disorienting. For most of us, these dramas show us the interaction between character—demonstrated (characterized) by the figures on the stage, the *dramatis personae*—and bad occasions/awful situations: Hamlet has to avenge the murder of his father.

The existence of so many different public usages for the word *tragic* suggested to me some blurring, overlapping of meanings. It seemed to me the journalistic usage *tragic* significantly skews the interrelationship of tragedy and trauma, where traumatizing events leave us with prolonged suffering. Tragedy has to do with what happens to us, as well as our response to that, a nexus or focus upon the boundary between outside impact and inside response and elaboration.

Projection

I figured that tragic process must have a beginning. Trying to locate the psychological origin of tragedy, I came to see that at the heart of theatrical drama is our capacity to *project* upon the outer world what we experience inwardly. Without *projection*, there is no drama, no theater; we cannot set up a stage to watch our story. Everything that is of current concern in our experience of drama is derived from this fundamental, and rather arduous, problematic fact of human existence. The major psychodynamic inquiries of the nineteenth and twentieth centuries, including Freud's, begin with projection as an essential part of their foundations of understanding of human nature.

Tragic literature provides the opportunity to focus exquisitely upon the boundary between inner and outer. We can view our inner experience, what it is and how it is projected upon the outer world. With tragedy, we can study the nature of projection and the pitfalls of its random, unmodulated, unacknowledged, and pervasive occurrence in our daily lives. The suffering tragic heroes and heroines endure is made visible through the mechanism of projection, and, it has been argued, by witnessing it in the theater, its perpetuative sting perhaps can be alleviated, bringing us to greater wisdom. Aeschylus' Oresteian chorus prays that good emerge from disaster.

Tragedy makes visible these implications of projection, especially its all-important *encapsulations*. The hero is encapsulated when he cannot break out of systems of values, or concepts of self. Encapsulations often lead to the kind of disasters that in the real world are commonly called tragic. In these situations, our sense of our boundaries is that they are fixed, without permeable ventilation. I realize that I am constitutionally sealed off from reality and other people when I project; I am victim and perpetrator of my deepest isolation.

Projection allows us to have all kinds of dramatic experience. *Hamlet*, Shakespeare's tragedy, demonstrates the dynamic of the projective phenomenon itself. Horatio is witness to Hamlet's progress and thus characterizes the heartbeat of projection. As audience, as we witness, we are like Horatio watching Hamlet, and thus observing, we may find a personal location beyond tragedy and the tragic. In this sense, Hamlet acts out what Horatio projects. Horatio : Hamlet :: audience : *Hamlet*. Tragedy, as a duchy in the kingdom of drama, focuses upon why drama occurs, as well as what its limits are.

Within the phenomenon of projection we can see a twofold function. As we project our inner life outward upon the world and upon other people, we may begin to sense that other people exist. They may take a role in our drama, or we in theirs. In this way, projection can be a developmental station on the way to empathic connection with the world beyond ourselves.

The other function of projection may be a response to some kind of inner system, a metaphysical, moral, epistemological, or psychological bag which we cannot punch ourselves out of, a pressurized inner encapsulation system, with oppositional boundaries we cannot enter or leave. Without such an internal obstructing system, would there be any need to transfer anything we experience about ourselves outside ourselves? Would we not do onto others what we would do unto ourselves? Or conversely, what we do unto ourselves, we do unto others; within projection, that is all we ever do.

Under the encapsulating, enshadowing blockade implied within the phenomenon of projection, our activities seem less significant, perhaps imitating something more "serious" because we do not experience ourselves as whole. We dwell in the dilemma "To be or not to be." With this focus, amid the cold and wet of England in late 1961, I was beginning to examine an issue that was to carry me into inner reaches of my psyche.

Dramatis Personae and Gestalt

The story and characters that appear on stage are a projection, an externalization, a dramatization, if you will, of our inner patterns of relationship and being. It was my brother who early on conveyed to me the insight that the *dramatis personae* are dramatic people, not just people people. We were discussing Nabokov's *Lolita,* which he thought described the integration, or lack of integration, of a single personality, including fragments called Humbert, Lolita, and the multifarious Quilty, not merely the outrageous story of a dirty old man. In like fashion the actors on stage embody portions of personality, making up a *gestalt,* a unified whole.

In gestalt theory, all parts of the story, dream, myth, whatever, can be witnessed as aspects of ourselves. In "Snow White and the Seven Dwarfs," Snow White encounters aspects of herself in the personae of the Seven Dwarfs, whom she learns to take care of. The principle can be extended so that all the characters, including the prince, the hunter, the wicked stepmother, the poison apple, even the deceased mother, are parts of our whole. How these fragments are connected into a unity, where the gestalt is revealed, is the main revelatory business of plot in drama and story.

Our tragic hero, such as Hamlet, which story-pattern we choose to represent on stage, runs into a snag, some division, some Grand Canyon in ourselves, expressed in activities which precipitate his, and our destruction. In the face of these difficulties, he moves along the rickety boundary of responsibility between inside and outside, revealing the dangers of arbitrarily determining that boundary and a resultant possible encapsulation of our spirit. In tragedy, the crucial interface between inside and outside has been distorted into a pattern.

As witnesses to the *pattern,* we can see the points at which boundaries (helpful) become encapsulations (not helpful) in people. Some encapsulation promulgates a pattern which takes narrative, story form. As theater spectators we are allowed to experience these patterns inwardly. Hopefully we create a safe space wherein to watch the patterns resolve, and energetic wholeness restored.

Studying various narratives, I came to see that the story itself might be unimportant to the resolution of an heroic pattern with its implied encapsulation. It seemed to me for this reason that Aristotle focused upon the structure of the plot and the necessity for plot as demonstrative gestalt to have a beginning, middle, and end. Thus we can focus upon what is rigid encapsulating pattern and what is flowing, energetic wholeness.

During each day, we rarely experience activities which bring us to a consistent, focused, and sustained sense of wholeness. In this way, our everyday activities may be seen as often random efforts to define ourselves and to express some underlying pattern that is intimately tied to our concept of self. Self, a formal proposal of identity, reflects the process by which our boundaries may become agents of encapsulation; we say, "This is me," or "This is not me."

It is possible to read Aristotle as challenging the very idea of self or personhood as we commonly understand that term. In this sense, tragedy does not occur to people, because most people act as fragments in process of assembly. Nor do we know easily how to achieve, for lack of a better term, wholeness.

People who think about these things note that we are usually selves *becoming*, not wholeness *being*. While tragedy may involve something impinging upon us, it can be seen not to occur to people because it is about what makes or does not make us think we are people. Tragedy in this sense happens within people.

Thus, dramatic tragedy is an *imitation* of life, an imitation of a *serious action*, not the same thing as imitating or representing people, who embody tragedy and are attempting to become selves or to be whole. If we encapsulate, we become fragments dwelling within an illusion of wholeness. Becoming a self suggests gaining admission to some club of wholeness, but *becoming* brings us up against fragmentations which paradoxically keep us encapsulated.

Perhaps for this reason, writers of tragedies came to be concerned with the gestalt, specifically through so-called unities of time, place and action. Each tragedy situation had to take place within the course of one day, in one place, describing one action.

What that action is, of course, is problematic, because mere activity, such as washing the dishes, for the most part does not define what action is. Action implies some integrity, or disintegrity, some relationship between the modes of becoming and of being. Implicitly, tragedians thus recognized the presence of fragmentation and encapsulation which needs witnessing, on its way to becoming a gestalt: *E pluribus unum.*

Scapegoating

After setting these tragic, difficult patterns out for examination, what do we do with them? We *scapegoat* them, which means we project some difficult and unpleasant aspect of ourselves onto someone else and then ritually cast them and, presumably, the badness they incarnate, out of town. Showing how if we rise in good fortune, we also fall, the hero/leader becomes a scapegoat, taking with him/her the difficult patterns that dwell within his community and, by extrapolation, within the members of the audience.

Our capacity to project, to identify with that projection, and to scapegoat are all aspects of the same epistemological phenomenon that makes tragedy tragic. And the recognition of the encapsulation of spirit which projection can imply is where the educational, preventative, and healing experience of tragedy begins; I intuited that this point of focus is where Freud began. Using this insight about projection, from a Western, Jewish sensibility, he proposed a vision of an alternative to suffering. For our culture, his lineage has raised the perhaps more eastern question, "Can we learn to distinguish between suffering, which might be avoidable or concludable, and pain, which might not?"

If we look for the conclusion of suffering in tragic drama, it most often appears to offer a superficial venue, wherein the tragically afflicted hero dies. This is an answer of some sort, that death ends our suffering, though afterlife visions of Christian hells and Tibetan bardos suggest even more arduous relationships possible between character and action and suffering there than here on earth. From a gestalt point of view, the hero/fragment, tyrannically characterized, dies, and wholeness may be restored to the entire personality, the tragic surround which survives after the heroic, fragmentary system disintegrates.

Somehow, in a best world, what is inner and what is outer could be well-delineated without our need for vigilance or for crossing a resistant boundary and placing our garbage on our neighbor's lawn and then blaming her/him for the mess. Christians would not have to blame Jews for the problem Jesus has left them with, nor do we have to scapegoat Mary Magdalene because we feel insecure or bad about ourselves.

Tragictatus

As a physician's son aware of the healing potential of viewing tragedic dramas, Aristotle terms "most tragic" (*tragictatus*) the non-extant tragedy *Cresphontes*, where a mother, Merope, who is about to kill a young man who is actually her son whom she thought dead, recognizes him as her son and does not kill him. Examining among others the plays of Aeschylus, Sophocles, and Euripides, I saw that the most tragic plays could be not just those plays that ended with the hero's death, or the wholesale slaughter of family or societal networks, but that tragedies as plays could describe some completion, some bottoming out process. Here, disasters arising from errors in projective identification are not fulfilled but avoided, in situations which most typical tragic playwrights do not envision, depict, or achieve.

Shakespeare certainly escorts us to some bottom. From the commonplace tragic understanding of wholesale disaster I think he can take us to the moment of *stasis* or immobility out of which healing movement can occur. Yet with the very significant exceptions of the late romances, he does not readily show us the healing moment of tragedy, which is not the same as taking us there. Perhaps that function is more often shown in his comedies.

His classical big tragedies (*Hamlet*, *Othello*, *King Lear*, *Macbeth*, and *Anthony and Cleopatra*) may give us primarily a sense of powers beyond human powers, of structured overwhelm, but not outright psychic anarchy. We are allowed only small, albeit significant glimpses of psychotic toxicity or true chaos; I think these can be glimpsed in the surround of formulations of power, the grotesque, and the sadistic. We are led to the bottom of human experience with no hope for completion, which itself is an emotional strategy or psychological placement from which our deepest movement, and healing, can occur.

I came to envision the goal of performed tragedy as ultimately resolving the relationship between character, action (*praxis*), and plot (the sequence of events or *muthos*), between *who* and what happens to that who, so the painful story would not have to be actually projected into real life, *i.e.*, acted out, by the members of the audience.

Experiencing *Oedipus Rex* in the theater, for example, we do not have to kill our fathers, marry our mothers, or put our eyes out. Rather, we can attend to a different, perhaps invisible level of action where such activities might originate. I was beginning to sense that we might have to experience the story in a different way than usual in order to be free of the pattern it tyrannically contains.

Tragedy is about something which happens to me, but also involves my response to the outside world. It describes catastrophe and its distorting impact upon the mindbody.

The challenge to fundamentalism that theater brings is significant. Even Freud had succumbed to a fundamentalist understanding of the myth in his rendering of the Oedipus complex. Yet at some intrapsychic, developmental level, the *pattern* contained within *Oedipus Rex* is what we have already experienced, or need to.

Somehow we can learn by the kinesthetic experience of the *narrative*, the combination of character, action, and plot, on the stage and so do not have to mirror it or act it out in our daily life. Yet we can safely experience the patterns that need completion, and by merely witnessing, the patterns can dissolve. We discover the patterns can dissolve without insisting they declare themselves only in narrative forms; they can be witnessed as *energetic*.

This is a capacity or lesson that the heroes in these dramas somehow do not "learn." Or their learning brings them face to face with narrative encapsulation, fostering the occasion to project. We project the pattern of our inner drama into story form—"Once upon

a time. . ."—and in the safety of the theater further project it outside
ourselves onto the stage. As student, I saw how we might begin to
witness the energetic and learn to stop our suffering, wherein our
energetic patterns are forever awaiting completion.

Bottoming Out

In our healing process, we intuitively know that there has to
be a *bottoming out* sequence where, hitting some nadir, everything
appears to be lost. Then occurs the turning where energetic
movement carries us out of being stuck, back to the surface. The
difference between, say, Shakespeare's *King Lear* and his *The
Winter's Tale* reflects these two phases of our healing process.

King Lear tells the story of an aging king who divides his
kingdom among his three daughters. His favorite, Cordelia, refuses
to obsequiously cater to his dotage vanity, and he banishes her. The
remaining two take over the now self-disempowered king, stripping
him of his attendant knights and trappings of royalty.

Unprotected on the heath by the accoutrements of ordinary
role sanity, there he endures the storm, external and internal, reminded
of his folly by the only retaining vestige of his royalty, his Fool. In this
moment he connects with his essential humanity, yet in the aftermath
of the demise of his entire kingdom, including activities of civil war
and grotesque violence, his good daughter is killed, and he himself
dies, broken. *King Lear* achieves the darkest absurdity and
nothingness from which later movement is possible, while *The
Winter's Tale* practically begins with a similar catastrophic
conclusiveness, then reveals how transformation and integrity are
gained.

In the second play, King Leontes in a fit of unfounded
jealously accuses his queen of infidelity with his best friend, plots to
kill him, orders his own infant daughter killed, and presumably causing
the death of his innocent wife, directly causes the death of his son,
who dies grieving the loss of his falsely accused mother. Realizing his
errors too late, the king dwells for fourteen years in penitential grief,

until the wise wife of one of his ministers helps restore wife, daughter, and friend to the humbled man.

To my understanding, *The Winter's Tale,* often characterized as a "romance," contains more significant information about this latter view of tragedy than *King Lear.* It fulfills the status of *tragictatus,* most tragic, because it ends relatively happily, having carried us to the tragic depths and revealed to us how the transition toward wholeness, or unity of time, place, and action, is achieved. In many people's estimation, as an ultimate tragedy, *King Lear* would come to mind first, because we think that anything that ends with such overwhelming, complex, absurd sadness qualifies as tragic.

In the Greek tradition, however, I sensed recognition of the necessity for balance and for witnessing change (*metabasis*) occurring within or as a *serious action* (*praxis*). In this Aristotelian definition, there is a difference between our human neurochemistry of activity and that of action. *Change* could mean any alteration, yet what tragic drama strives to evoke is closer to what we call a "sea change," wherein the entire relationship of our personality to something as elemental as gravity shifts. Without explaining myself fully at this point, I think *serious action* is that which is not made in reference to or motivated by traumatic patterning, either within our self, or in the culture without.

Where is the Starting Point of Suffering?

More important, by attempting to conclude suffering, tragic drama poses the question: Where is the starting point of suffering? Since before Aristotle, the examination of tragic theory has sought answers to this question by focusing upon energetics with the following logic:

Where do these self-destructive patterns begin? Do they begin with our environment, our community, which instills destructive attitudes and experiences, with our heredity, or the gods? Could they start with the spirit, which is perceived within our human experience as *energy* or the source of energy? Where does the energy of our *mindbody* reside, how can it be viewed, how does that energy manifest in patterns of personality, intention, and action, and how are they transmuted? These are central questions of tragic literature and tragic experience.

All tragic theorists are moralists in the English usage of the word *moral*. Morality is not superficially asking questions about right and wrong activities such as "Is abortion right or wrong?" Rather, moral questions more subtly may pose the problem, "From what position(s) do I view, or apparently choose to view, ultimate reality, and how does that positioning determine what I see or experience or appear to choose?" Again, the essential problem morality addresses involves projection and how we connect with reality.

Presumably, subsequent and righteous, *i.e.*, moral, action can be derived from our positioning, including our relationship to ultimate reality, sometimes called God. Using as examples the plays of Sophocles, Aeschylus, Racine, or, say, Arthur Miller, as moralists, tragic theorists help us position ourselves for viewing an otherwise fluctuating, often unmanageable series of occasions in what we might call experience, a reality that includes impossible, inevitable destructions.

In tragic drama, the relationship of character to plot shows these patterns taking hold in such a way that the relationship between what a character does, and who s/he thinks s/he is, is seriously juxtaposed, compromised, and ultimately revised. Oedipus hunts to banish the murderer of his father and discovers it is himself he banishes.

In tragedy there is a reversal *(peripeteia)* of, for lack of a better term, vector, or trajectory of fate. In this sense the origins of suffering are revealed as contained in an inflexible adherence to some personality-attenuated narrative. This adherence is somehow irrelevant to serious action, which somehow involves change *(metabasis)*, which overcomes the hero(ine). Often we are thrust even beyond the easy answer that death is where we can see that change. Witnessing tragedies, we move beyond death as change, to the serious action beyond ordinary activity which generates change and propels us to a revised experience of what we are.

Reading *Emma*

In England in the early 1960s, I studied among many others Ibsen, Shaw, Conrad, Hobbes, Hooker, Bacon, and Jane Austen. With the respectful support of my professors and fellow students, as well as the experience of mobilizing energies to stay warm and dry during uncommonly cold, damp, and dark winters which may have promulgated some seasonal affective disorder, I came into a series of insights about the nature of tragedy which I dared apply to myself.

I was examining Queenie Leavis's proposal that all of Jane Austen's novels are, in effect, the same story, stacked in outline form in Jane Austen's desk drawer from the beginning of her career as a writer. Each novel she completed is a duplicate of the prior one, only, in each successive novel she finished, Jane Austen drew closer to a fundamental "problem" containing a pattern, which, as a woman of the late eighteenth century, she confronted. Using Leavis's strategy, I thought it had to do with the relationship between men and women, and in particular, with marriage: What was she doing without a husband? The problem is stated obversely in the opening line of *Pride and Prejudice*:

> It is a truth universally acknowledged that a single man in possession of a good fortune must be in want of a wife.

Jane Austen's exploration into the relationships of men and women leading to marriage begins with the somewhat adolescent satire *Northanger Abbey* and gains force with *Sense and Sensibility*, winding through recapitulations of the patterns permeating this issue in *Pride and Prejudice*. The first versions of these three novels are written between 1795 and 1798, and *Pride and Prejudice* is published in 1813. She appears to uncover a complex, depressed core in the mannerist *Mansfield Park*, completed in 1814.

With a sense of real excitement, I garnered that Jane Austen writes her most complete vision of a tragic crisis in *Emma* (1815); and I was not alone in intuiting that something intense, even of a cutting edge, goes out of her brilliant writing after *Emma*. It appears she hovers in the aftermath of her effort with the partially completed, softer *Persuasion*, published posthumously, and her final fragment, *Sanditon*, which contains echoes of her earlier, unedited and untempered patterns.

Emma seemed to me the highest expression of Jane Austen's art, an extraordinary, satiric, and ultimately deeply sensed examination of the dangers of projective identification, which I perceived lies at the root of tragedy. To put it currently and a bit heavily, *Emma* might be seen as a comic commentary upon a barely avoidable toxicity of our fundamental, perhaps constitutional narcissistic encapsulation.

Her mother having died early on, Emma Woodhouse, an intelligent and accomplished young gentlewoman of twenty, has been raised by her governess Miss Taylor, and when Miss Taylor leaves to get married, Emma is left the mistress of the house, living with her comically dotty, self-absorbed, and rigid father.

Perhaps with an unchallenged cleverness, and full of youthful judgment, Emma takes on a pretty, seventeen year-old "protégé," Harriet Smith. Harriet embodies a less accomplished, slower-paced energy not of the mind, but of the heart, an energy nexus which in some fundamental way Emma has ignored, brought up as she was within the pressure of her father's self-preoccupation.

Prone to seeking to control everyone's social business, and elegantly cautioned not to by her perspicacious somewhat older friend Mr. Knightley, Emma unwittingly projects onto Harriet feelings for Mr. Knightley, pushing the simpler woman in his direction, with almost disastrous emotional results for Harriet, Harriet's future husband Robert, Knightley, and ultimately for herself.

Emma finally comes to a recognition or *anagnōrisis*, that it is she, Emma, who must marry Knightley, her thoughtful Horatio-like confidant who witnesses her with honesty and understanding. Emma's sense of shame at having encouraged Harriet to believe it was she, not Emma, whom Mr. Knightley was destined to marry, is profound:

> ... to see that Harriet's hopes had been entirely groundless, a mistake, a delusion, as complete a delusion as any of her own—that Harriet was nothing; that she [Emma] was everything herself; that what she had been saying relative to Harriet had been all taken as the language of her own feelings; and that her agitation, her doubts, her reluctance, her discouragement, had been all received as discouragement for herself.

> How to do the best by Harriet was of more difficult decision; how to spare her from any unnecessary pain; how to make her any possible atonement; how to appear least her enemy? On these subjects her perplexity and distress were very great—and her mind had to pass again and again through every bitter reproach and sorrowful regret that had ever surrounded it.

It is a brief bottoming out experience, and we are spared some of its heavy burden. Yet the convincing, happy resolution of this emotional conundrum underscores how little we know about ourselves and how hard it is to know others. And more penetratingly, because of projection and its corollary, the underlying, easy potential for an enthralling encapsulation, we witness with consistent focus how little we can know: How much effort and luck it takes to see and be seen by ourselves and those around us. As I read it then, I felt *Emma*, like the story of Merope, fulfilled the most tragic (*tragictatus*) status identified by Aristotle, namely showing the avoidance of actual consequences of the perpetration of some bad pattern projected upon others.

The goal of tragedy, staged and written, can be seen to be using projective identification in order *not* to have disaster. Tragic narratives rather induce resolutions of the patterns the story contains so that they may be fundamentally and developmentally safely completed. We spectators are freed of having to act the patterns out, setting them into narrative, correcting the mistaken judgment (*hamartia*) that that was the only way to discharge them. We do not have to move with often disastrous activity in order to experience the movement of serious action.

Jane Austen's Relationship to Her Novels

The most tragic forms within narratives reveal that suffering is based upon illusion which does not have to be perpetrated; and perpetration is not the way out of suffering. This means not confusing a part for the whole, a character fragment for the unity of personality, and the resultant attempt to project these fractionations outward. In summary, for Aristotle, *tragictatus* implies human mastery of vectors at the source of suffering.

The insight I strongly came to then was that Jane Austen bore the same relationship to her novels as Emma did to Harriet. As novelist, she was urging forward toward the reader an immense charm and brilliant accomplishment which was being exposed finally as surrogate, at the expense of Jane Austen's heart. Sadly, perhaps her heart had been prematurely affected by the death of a young clergyman she may have loved. The details and impact of her involvement are important and unknown.

Shortly after she comes to her clearest realization about projection in *Emma*, published in 1815, it seemed to me that a corollary begins to work itself out. Neither her novels nor the personae contained within them can "marry," for marriage implies a complicated combination of a social and personal, supra-literary, supra-artistic relationship. Jane Austen herself, now a maiden aunt of nearly four decades, must marry, or cannot. The pattern she is trying to complete becomes, in *Emma*, visible and impossible, and within two years of its publication, in 1817, she dies of Addison's disease, having partially finished only *Persuasion*, with sections of *Sanditon* remaining to give us a sense of how in turn each work was brought forward.

Jane Austen was perhaps too wise and clever, too ironic as well as dear, to find a man suitable for her. Who can say? Her early *Lady Susan* suggests her examining a vision of ambition, judgment, and vanity which she chose not to approach as directly in her heroines in subsequent works except in *Emma*. But the encapsulation that she describes in *Emma* is so poignant, so profoundly comically and morally rendered, that when I first read the novel in England, I felt compelled to turn the whole projective formulation upon myself, perpetrating a crisis that led me into psychoanalysis, then the most established self-examination game in town.

CHAPTER ONE: MORE JOURNEY

My Own Tragic Patterning

Basically, my question for myself was, "How was I, in my early twenties, through books and studies and my intense and academic involvement with ideas, keeping myself away from my own involvement with people and with myself, in personal and intimate ways?" By discussing books, and tragic theory, and the like, how, like Emma and her creator, was I avoiding my own projectivity, encapsulation, and ultimately tragic patterning? By this I did not mean that I had been placed particularly *in extremis* by life; I ran what many would think was a privileged course.

But facing my own personal patterning and, in spite of a long-standing maternal and paternal family lineage which selectively supported introspection, I sought to root out the source of the suffering my patterning now entailed by looking into an over-the-shoulder mirror of my own capacity to project and be projected upon; in so doing, I felt the frightening weight of tragic awareness.

What I had thought was normal and ordinary in me, including a profile of truncated social intimacy, now became oppressive. The volume on my sexual and spiritual preoccupations increased, as well as an irrational conviction about the impossibility of expressing them in acceptable ways. Believing as I did that tragedy was about moral perspective as well as the sometimes dire events that shaped that perspective, I did not need a new Titanic, Hiroshima, or a new Holocaust to place me in the problem.

Those histories, the last significantly, had already given me a sense of imperative, or perhaps better, a lack of imperative: That I could no longer unmindfully sustain the cultural *status quo* within which I had been raised. As a young boy, hearing about Hiroshima, the Japanese war-prisons, and the German concentration camps, some youthful allegiance to or trust in all, not just Axis, authority systems passed out of me, dovetailing with a growing awareness of the adult world's human compromises, self-betrayals, and impactions.

Immersed as they were in tragedies in all senses of the word, in some ways people who endured traumatizing, horrible events might not be able initially to adumbrate the issues of tragedy. In the sense I was pursuing, tragedies are about witnessing the true, severe limitations of perception and action for everyone, not just for those severely afflicted or victimized by these limitations.

The inner work I was attempting did not deny the reality of the cataclysm, but at some preventive level, I sought to limit the scale of tragic enactment which ended in situations like the Holocaust by looking for its point of origin, which might be visible in the simplest, most minor, even Austenian, moments. Looking amid the ordinariness of the problems which lead to tragedy, I felt supported by the insights of Hannah Arendt and Georges Bataille, among others.

If I could learn how to eliminate the now preoccupying patterning within myself, and master projection within and without my self, I might be able to change at the deepest levels and to live a life *tragictatus*, sharing that safe and basically conflict-resolving vision with others. I did not see quite how I was going to extend that learning into the world—perhaps through teaching or writing. During those weeks and months, often it seemed that though now I had my hand near, even on, a somewhat random tiller of self-examination, I was being carried by an energetic wind which drove me into the depths, where in fact I longed to be, as well as near dangerous shoals.

To understand that we project aspects of ourselves onto the world beyond us and specifically onto people and situations outside ourselves can bring a cold wind upon the sunny innocence of childhood and adolescence. As I then perceived it, projection is *the* primary psychological and social fact, and the scapegoating errors we make under its spell are at the base of tragic experience. I too was the tragedy I was studying. I embodied some tragic, encapsulated and encapsulating patterning within myself.

Diving into this sea, I began to sense the fragmentations within my own personality which heretofore I had avoided. I felt I was irrationally dwelling upon certain idea systems and yet was not able to sense their impact in my daily life. I knew the ideas and situations I studied were ultimately about me and what was potential within me, but at some level, intellectually facile as I had become, I could not connect them to my actual behavior. Longing for the intimacy of a permanent commitment to another person, I somehow could not establish one. Even my initial attempts threw me back upon myself.

When twenty-two, I returned to New Jersey for the Christmas holiday, and my father played for me a tape recording of my thirteenth birthday, complete with the sounds of my by now dead grandmother's voice and those of my family. I was overwhelmed. At some preverbal level, I heard in the resonances of my thirteen year-old voice patterns which had not moved in the subsequent nine years of my life, and I sensed being ultimately trapped by some force I could not put words to, not knowing how to extract myself.

Returning to England, I felt increasingly absorbed in this process and alienated from the support of kinder forces in the world. When initially I discussed with one of my Cambridge dons what I thought I was trying to do, he advised me with English decorum, and perhaps wisdom, "We think it best not to apply such academic subjects to oneself personally."

American *naïf* that I was, I assumed that anything short of applying my ideas to my experience compromised my integrity, something I felt I could not do. Preoccupied with images of tenderness and unfulfillable desire for connection, my long-present inner pressures toward intimacy were no longer deniable, and so alone, day by day, I ventured into a place of existential and deeply felt, irreconcilable despair.

Like Lucifer, the angel closest to God, I witnessed a terrifying division within myself and a related encapsulation from the outside world, a Hell in which I would never be connected to what I intuited was ultimate reality. The pain of this sequence was intolerable, and I wanted to die, soon. I knew suicide was very possible.

In the rush of energy and toxicity which these recognitions released, I felt disoriented within, not in control in the old familiar ways. With the kind support of my brother, returning to Yale University for graduate studies, I moved quickly to establish myself in a psychoanalytic relationship, stabilizing my situation and trying to continue my search.

From High Station to Low

Aristotle has described an audience's response to tragic drama and the fate of its hero, who plummets from high station to low, from good fortune to bad, as involving a sequence of pity and fear. Following his lead, I reasoned that members of a theater audience watching a tragedy begin by experiencing pity for the fallen tragic hero and then experience fear, because they realize that if they can experience the pattern enacted outside themselves, then on some level they must hold the same pattern potential within themselves.

I myself had traversed this sequence at a performance of Stravinsky's *Oedipus Rex*, wherein the terror I felt was visceral. What is recognizable outside ourself reverts to possibility within the so-called boundaries of our so-called self. This sequence seemed to me a description of what on some new level I was experiencing. For the first time in my adult life, I felt seriously, radically, spiritually afraid, and no matter what I thought, my fear would not go away.

The characters and plot of tragic drama are a projection (a scapegoat?) of some otherwise difficult to perceive pattern in ourselves which is projected outward upon the stage in artistic form. There it has the capacity to induce a deep cleansing of emotion and perhaps lead to transformation, both individual and social. Such *katharsis* leads us to what I would now call *right action*, a movement free of the encumbrances of plot and character.

Aristotle recognized that there was a "serious action" (*praxis*) which the drama imitated, and I saw that the serious action was, in some quite literal way, in the head and psyche of the spectator. What was on stage represented some important pattern, cognitive, emotional, and ultimately energetic in the minds of the spectators. Even in the early 1960s, I perceived the energetic realm as the point of origin of character and narrative.

It was only after years of searching at this level that I confirmed how our patterns imitated in so-called character and plot are non-verbal, chemical, and traumatically held at *subtle energy* levels. Scientifically controversial, subtle energies are thought to include hierarchies of the electro-magnetic aurae which surround and interpenetrate the visible human body, and, according to strategists, control and densify or *incarnate* into molecules, cells, and tissues, and emotions. Or at least, I came to intuit, these levels are the final frontiers from which my patterns could be best viewed and appreciated, and ultimately transformed.

The nineteenth and early twentieth century preoccupations with what critics have called *mimēsis* (imitation) in some ways had begged this question. What if the action that was being imitated in art, and in particular tragic drama, was invisible, and beyond the thought and speech centers of the brain? Freud had posited the unconscious as the "place" where such patterns might reside, but too often what those of us involved in psychoanalysis did was to remain in ideational thought, "in the mental head," as if that were the best, most accurate place to watch the psychic fireworks, and, presumably, their origin. Only gradually did I come to understand the risks involved in manifesting this bias, which I thought I had practiced enthusiastically for years.

Psychoanalytic modes kept to the cognitive shore, reefing our sails with interpretation, not moving into silence, mystery, and letting go. For me and the others with whom I discussed my process, it was all talk and some feeling, but only on the part of the analysand, not the analyst really. His connection to his client is often intentionally obscured.

How to get to the heart of the issues and placate the forces and drives which were coursing through me? My work on tragedy and on myself through psychoanalysis interwove. In analysis, the activity was talk as the way to appropriate the patterning, the tragic form. What, however, if Aristotle's serious action began not with a movement, but with an immobility, a lack of movement which our brain continuously scans for until the pattern is dissolved and the energy set in motion again? Talk, or even thought, might not help.

What if the very idea of imitation places us on the field of what is now called *dissociation* (*cf.* Chapter One), seriously challenging our ideas about the origins of art and literature? Could their patterns be based upon some energetic illusion which was not necessary? The importance of these insights also etched itself into my plate only gradually, over decades.

Now a young man of twenty-three, I was dissatisfied with myself in profound ways. Beyond intellect and sensibility, I did not know how to transform. I felt I was on a trajectory that was leading me beyond my capacity to understand, and so I had to take this problem and make it my own—in short, take responsibility. Three ways to continue my examination of these issues were through study, introspection, and relationships.

Psychoanalysis

As a graduate student, however, I was faced with the problem of my own brain and its functioning. How could I see its tragic patterns, much less even hope to do something with them? Psychoanalysis then had seemed the only creditable modality, and it specifically addressed projection in its recognition of *transference*, where the client projects his inner drama upon his relationship with the analyst. I continued for four years of talk and "free-association," flat on my back facing the tiled office ceiling of a cold, analytic hardliner, whom I thought I respected, though not necessarily warmed to.

My analyst had initially identified my pattern of taking on everything, asking me, "Do you have to do all the work?" In the context of initial interviews, I was reduced to unusual tears by the apparent empathy of his question, and I thought he knew what was up with me in a way other analysts I interviewed had not. In some odd way, this was the first and perhaps last empathic statement I felt he made in four years of our interaction.

In England, my goal had been to get to the bottom of things by studying as I saw it, the deepest and heaviest tradition in the humanities. Amid the growing cultural crisis of the 1960s, thick with pervasive, virtually omnipresent projective tragic patterning, I attempted to walk my talk. Desperate and intense, I kept finding unavoidable examples of projection everywhere, with few people attending to this phenomenon in themselves. With brief forays into essential, non-projective contact, however, *I* was turning into the bottom of things, often crawling through day and night, grateful if I could achieve even a reptilian fogginess.

Tragedy had to do with rock-bottom suffering, necessary and avoidable, and within the tragic tradition I saw my own interest gain focus. What would it take to lift off the curse of self-imprisonment which the men and women around me were mindlessly perpetuating? And as a young, sensitive adult with a disembodied intellect, I was only beginning to see, with horror, how much I could resemble them.

As a child and more intensely into my young adulthood, I was deeply troubled, embarrassed, and constricted by adults' behavior and their presentations of self. Not that some engaged me without depth; often I was challenged by them, a distinctive number of them in very kind, very important ways, including, critically, my parents. I was not as available to instruction as I liked to think I was, and I received real, distinctive support from some members of the adult world, including my parents and my family.

I received as well from adults other things not so pleasant, present, or connected. But what I sensed and knew was true about them, particularly their suffering, did not make it easy to keep myself focused on my own patterning, nor were any of them prepared to help me remove these patterns in myself. Generally, they wanted to administer an easy lesson, easily learned, which included adjustment and accommodation to the demands of the outer world.

At their schools, churches, parties, in conversations, I encountered an underlying despair anchoring an often shallowly-expressed or compacted existence. I felt they needed me to be OK, even when I was not. Whether this was actually true or part of the pattern I was perpetrating was another matter. I could not easily extract myself from them.

My Views of My Sexuality

Even as an adolescent, I had felt the missing link in the chain of people's integrity was sexual, for sexuality seemed forbidden, a realm of conflict and of truth for practically everybody. In my own case my sexuality seemed to put me directly in connection with my touching, passionate, and loving self, yet a self for some reason I only obliquely, rarely shared. Given its compassionate, passionate, and tender nature, as I experienced it from within, how could that inner, omni-present reality be a mistake?

My experience with my parents and family gave me confidence about my abilities to bring pleasure and depth from an early age, and I began to express profound longings for connection with both boys and girls right from the start of kindergarten. I treasured the intimacies of childhood and was troubled to the point of being overwhelmed when I could not experience them. I did not understand the sadism, the hostility, and the suffering which I witnessed, particularly in those families I knew, and I felt angry, frightened, and helpless about all that. I suppose my frustration could be framed that I was one of those who, given such choice, would rather kiss than kill.

From my earliest memories, I had an active sensuality which became increasingly problematic as I ran into other people's fears as well as my precocious sexuality. Even casual happy connections quickly escalated in my imagination to marriage with classmates, teachers, and friends. I did not experience a latency period, nor any time before that could I be characterized as sensually, erotically dormant, though I pretty much kept my hands to myself, with two exceptions.

For the first seven years of grade school, and after, I sustained one consistent, deep, and loving relationship with my girl friend, to whom in my imagination I was married, and which intermittently expanded into a love triangle with a boy friend. I would openly kiss them in school and out, in plain view of everybody, until I was ridiculed for it and learned how to suppress my activity. I recall puzzling at the age of six how as a grown-up was I going to bring these two parts of my affections together.

As I moved into adolescence and young adulthood, I ran into a can of worms. My internally perceived desire for physical, sexual closeness, universal, polymorphous, omnipresent, passionate, and attractive, was actually overlaid with interlocking images of libidinal freedom in patterns whose intensity and repetition indicated addiction, not choice. My interior experience was of pressure which could be responded to only problematically. There was no unobstructed opening for expression of love for me that I could envision. I could not hold and kiss the people who moved me.

I would respond to others by sensing their fluidity, then I locked into focus upon where they could not move, their held places, their suffering. I longed to join them in the interface between their flow and their holding, somehow imagining resolutions of the holding into a flow. This was my first and radically endured experience of the healing drive in eros.

My sexual fantasies were full of passion and tenderness, marked by parallel confidence-sharing and playful overcoming of inconsequentialities. They had a sense of moment, sufficiency, and also of being. The world I encountered within myself and without was that this vision was only rarely achieved, and more likely than not, restricted by society, which provided no visual demonstration of these possibilities.

Movies and books rarely combined discourse with intercourse, and the pornography I saw hinted at this ecstatic, boundaried, uninhibited sharing, but generally objectified a frozen formulaic energy which did not reveal the essence or how I could achieve it. Its fetid moves were urgent, rather than contemplative and sequential, and often I was left responding to its urgency but somehow feeling self-deserted. Though a significant release, my masturbation seemed only a constricted prelude to something greater, a something which was not just sexual or even relational. I sensed the healing potential in sexual experience but did not experience it.

My forced, defensive imposition of this topic at college had brought criticism from perhaps equally conflicted classmates. I could see their inhibitions and defenses, and my own, but I was powerless to do anything about mine, or theirs, whose suffering disturbed me as much as my own. My needs for human contact, profound and demanding, were set against a repressive internal and external environment. As a graduate student in foggy, damp, cold England, what I had seen in Jane Austen applied to myself: I needed to connect not through books and ideas, but directly, sensately, and with people.

I left analysis four years later with very few of my patterns assailed or transformed. My analyst seemed powerless to assist me, nor did he seem to want to. Being a good analysand, I agreed with his abandoning strategy as a sign that I was in transference, a strategy easy to understand intellectually, but hard to do anything about. When I wasn't sensating, I sensed I needed more distance, less passion.

Within this rubric, some significant inroads were made in terms of direct connection with other, important individuals. In fits and starts, I began deep, intense connections with men and women, including with the woman who was to become my wife. But these achievements with friends and lovers seemed opposed by analytic process; they were made surreptitiously against the opacity of cold-turkey psychoanalytic modeling. And they were slight, compared with my inner process which would not be stilled, feeding as it did upon intellectual ideation.

Perhaps I was too familiar with Freud and Jung already, too eager to develop insight, or too defensive in applying insight, too much in the verbal, cognitive, analytic centers of my brain, too intellectually defended, for more of the same to do any good. Certainly my rigidities were more profound than I realized, and for many years I blamed myself for whatever stalemate or failure my attempts at psychoanalysis entailed.   So eager to make the psychoanalysis work, at times I felt I must not have even entered it, and that if pushed, my analyst would reply coolly about me, "But when is he going to start?"

In fact, I had given psychoanalysis a good run, as good as many associates about whose analyses I heard. It had preoccupied me, and yet it had not helped me to resolve my preoccupations about sexuality and intimacy. I had been raised in spiritual, Protestant religious disciplines in which the default position was to take individual responsibility as much as possible. I was left with taking responsibility for a sense of contactlessness with the analyst which was counter to my deepest instincts, knowledge, and intuition. I ended up stabilizing my process and doing all the work and not really learning how not to.

My Father

One basic problem that had moved me all these years probably boiled down to my frustration with my father's toxic patterns, which, though externally successful in many ways, he struggled throughout his life to master.

As a young child, I had fallen in love with both my mother and my father, imitating their ways, their attitudes, their manner of holding themselves in their bodies, their emotional and cognitive gestures, their beliefs, and their integrities. And they reflected back that adoration, giving me support and encouragement, respect and engagement. I fed upon a very rich broth, which continues to stand as a model for me.

I basked in the admiration my father engendered as a man of intelligence and humor, successful in his business and in the world. He was so interesting, so imaginatively captivating, so funny and verbally measured, that I could not keep away from him. I found his eccentricities charming and distinctive, and I came to value them and those of his friends and acquaintances, above ordinary ways of being social, which to my discriminating sensibility soon became conventional.

My father would come to tuck us in at night and give us delicate backrubs, telling us stories with his words and fingers which were transporting, though because of his predisposition to narcolepsy, as children we would soon have to push the snoring giant out of our beds so we, not he, could sleep. I swallowed him whole, as I had my mother, though she in a different way.

As a pre-adolescent, I watched my father step carefully, insightfully, through the suburban New Jersey paranoia clustering around Adlai Stevenson, and the McCarthy hearings, and I came to depend upon his liberal, intricate formulations interpreting the events and issues of the day. It was only later in our lives that I sensed his conservatism, perhaps his unrationalized fear, emerge, while I was left holding the liberal, expansionist, exploratory bag of life he had earlier proclaimed and valued.

I attended an all-male preparatory country day school, where the lessons of isolation of male adolescence were instilled with daily brutality. I entered Yale, my father's college, which had become a central part of his identity as one of its very active alumni. Yale was to deepen our connection, and, as I strategized with college admissions officers, by entering it, my choice of Yale also was to allow me to separate out successfully from my father, facing the giant, while presumably taking the best of that tradition that had appeared to give so much to him.

In fact, it was while at Yale I began to experience the discrepancy between my father's reality and my own, a painful contrast, in spite of his sustained interest in the changing profile of college life. In New Haven I initiated a movement out from under a shadow which Yale as an ethos cast upon all my family members' lives.

By the time of my graduate studies and my psychoanalysis there, our contacts were vigorous, but also strained, as my father could not follow the direction I was taking as readily as he perhaps wanted to. In many senses, I was moving into an academic, creative, introspective career which he desired for himself.

He wanted me to report what my psychoanalysis, which he supported financially, was showing me as a way to help his own understanding. He also sabotaged that effort by disparaging it; some part of him did not want it to work. He would joke that, short of my converting to confessional Catholicism, we should get onto the couch together. I would remind him that in all probability he would fall asleep, and I would be left talking. During one confrontation as I was getting out of my parents' car on New Haven's Elm Street, I finally stated that his Yale and mine were two different experiences, and his anguished response was, "No, they are not, because you and I are the same."

I was as troubled as he by the gap between us, yet I felt I had to establish some boundary, if only instinctively, to protect my own development and not be swept into his encompassing, complicated emotional embrace. He wanted me happy in the same way he was happy, and, I suppose, to be unhappy in the way he was unhappy.

When I was not following the life path as he knew it, he felt hurt and, I think, a curious sense of personal betrayal, as well as depressive isolation. I had seen his suffering, which could not be assuaged by being a man at Yale, nor the life it had proposed. Like many men of his roaring twenties pre-Depression generation, he appeared to dig into the banana, certainly farther than many, and then to swallow the remainder of his imprisonment whole.

He was in some essential way right about our being the same, but not in the details, nor in his continuing attempts to appropriate my reality. I could not share my sensuous life with him, though the adventures I took in therapeutic modalities were prefigured in his own

post-graduate adult education, particularly his study of General
Semantics with Alfred Korzybski.

The violation I felt when near him I knew was a projective
communication of his own inner process, and it was countered by my
desire to hold onto the early glow of our connection which had
sustained me during my early years growing up. I think I would have
liked nothing better than to please him by joining his world, if I could
have, if in some deep conspiratorial way he had not made it clear what
cost membership in that world entailed.

But I could not fit the mold he desired, in part because his
world did not ultimately help him with his private patterns of
suffering, which included his need to overwhelm and shape the
experience of others. All of that was exercised from within his
heartfelt desire to share.

For diverse people living at arm's length, he could be superb;
for those of us closest to his patterns, it was often another matter.
Yale, for all his giving to its community with intelligence and
creativity, could not contain my father's patterns, and thus became
pivotal in a dynamic of avoidance, rather than just a strength. It was
hard to talk with him about anything else.

The older he and I got, the more difficult and uniform the
exchanges, though there was an intensity and richness that friends
hearing about them envied. My father was jealous and possessive of
me, yet critical and stymieing when in discussion, revealing a
competitive and judgmental streak which juxtaposed sharply with his
wide-ranging intellect and his caring. It was hard to have so much
with him and still be left wondering.

He continued with whimsical irony to play on the piano an old
revenge-for-a-broken-heart song, "It's all the same to me, whether
you go or stay." Though perhaps his intention was satirical, the
rhythm of his longing for connection and denial of its impact which the
song expresses has helped shape my experience of adult male life to
the present day. That was a problematic side of a glowing social
presence and imaginative paterfamilias for hundreds of people.

Perhaps we were mutually disappointed by each other's failures. His suffering, and my attempts to rescue him, and he me, and in response to which activities he continually offered up his self-abuse in the form of criticizing and yes-butting me, and our mutual failure, all motivated me to keep asking the question, "Yes, you talk one way, but your interactions, your body, your eyes, reveal a different text."

A Different Text

In fact, this was a variant "lyric" he often "sang" himself, as he commented upon, often with humorous accuracy and telling, ultimately humane vision, the processes of his family, college classmates, and friends around him. When I would confront him or his college reunion cronies, I would usually get denial that they had been distributing their suffering in my direction, or that I was incorrect for sensing their pain, which I felt viscerally when with them. I had picked up my father's very own battleflag, and when I looked back to see where he was, I found him looking in another direction or asleep.

Of course his friends were not dumping their pain in the standard way of crying into their beers, though they sometimes did that with me. When they came into the room, or talked about their experience, few revealed directly how far from integrity of spirit they felt. Yet in different ways they all expressed the importance of that objective to themselves, either directly, or indirectly by implication and use of their bodies (many drank heavily). What I experienced was their imprisonment, and I longed to share and see their balance restored, and in some remarkable cases did so. With men and women, I wanted to see and be seen without encapsulating shadows, face to face, even body to body, soul with soul.

I was unable to break through my father's encapsulations, which I know privately bothered him as much as they bothered me. In his sleep, he would groan and shout with nightmares, only to awaken startled and confused, denying that anything had troubled him.

His most pernicious and pervasive private pattern was denial, of the addictive way he related to his children and denial of his dependency upon others. He would refuse to buckle his seat belt when I drove the car for him, even though I expressed my deep concern for his safety. Typically, he would play solitaire while conversing with me. At one point late in his life, I said, "I am sick and tired of your denials; they don't work for me."

"Well," he responded, "they work for me."

A funny, intelligent, sensitive and shy, big and impacted, self-styled "angular" man (his was a forceps delivery), loved by many, he died in the late 1980s, giving me as the last of many rich, often juxtaposing and provocative gifts, the impression of his not having learned how to settle the major patterns of suffering of his life. Why was that impression so absolute, so radical? More vigilant than most people about the deceptions of language for definition of self, he ultimately succumbed to its hollow enthrallments as his patterns of toxicity would not leave by command alone. And in this, I think, he was not the only one among men of his generation.

My mother and I may disagree now about the extent to which my father did not resolve his traumata, and we approach our opinions of him from different points of view; I was his son, not his wife.

My mother reports that she experienced his capacity for intimacy and imaginative understanding as warm and unusual. Not without conflict, she felt his relationship with her was characterized by mutual devotion, and that the meaning they found and created there exemplified their creative expectations for marriage.

Challenged and loyally supported by her, toward the end of his life, he told me, "As far as you children go, my personal emotional priority is with your mother." I recall recognizing the truth of this and liking his clarity. And particularly at the end, perhaps he had resolved some issues of suffering and isolation within their relationship.

I also know that the sense of finality he gave me at the end was real and was what I now understand to be a phase of resolution of holding patterns. At the place of traumatic holding, there is no movement nor can there be, no matter what changes have been made elsewhere in our personality and our chemistry. When couples argue at this level, the spouse says, "You never tell the truth!" whether the other does or not. At the level of traumatic holding, which is what matters to brain, our impaction is eternal.

How this lineage of trauma is transmitted, between father and son, parent and child, became my question and at times my rage. After years of coming to the surface if merely to breathe, my only answer then was that it was an invisible, choiceless transmission, occurring at a level that had rendered us Chekovianly immobilized.

All the holding was transferred through a medium or at a level that could not be observed. Only indirectly appropriated, beyond language and symbol, the patterns were not seen at their point of origin, hence their hapless recurrence, without intention, consideration, or reflection.

I was standing at the stern of a boat watching its wake without being able to see how the boat created it. In marriage we may be given the opportunity to confront trauma in ourselves and in those we marry, but in the blood-gene connection, for the child there may be a deeper healing imperative.

It has taken me years to glimpse beyond the haplessness of it all, which my father painfully showed me, to see the superficiality of discernment about these patterns which had kept me from real knowledge. And that this issue, as my father's son, was what I needed to explore.

After Psychoanalysis

Following psychoanalysis, each turn in my work led to deeper connection with my patterns. In the late 1960s and early 1970s, I kept exploring various therapeutic and self-education modalities, trying to unlock the basic story that would lead to recognition of an underlying pattern, which, in effect, would result in direct perception of some primary (serious) action or immobility. Somehow its lifting off would result in deeper, cleaner experience, not the toxic densities of the suburban American East Coast culture with which I had problematically grown up. I began as a counselor, teacher, and lecturer, setting up interactions with undergraduates, and later, graduate students and clients which were direct, confrontational, and personal.

I became a freelance therapist, studying energetic strategies of Wilhelm Reich, to me a most creative elaborator and extender of Freudian insight. Yet, no matter how far from the mainstream I ventured, at each point I ran into peers and experts alike who were projecting and perpetrating unresolved, perhaps unresolvable patterns upon clients and friends. I was always left with the question, "Yes, you talk one way, but your actions and your body say something, completely, appositely different." Again, I found this apperception exquisitely and pervasively painful.

I hoped body workers would provide new, clear examples of integrity, yet with some exceptions, the characteristic moment they too were moving toward seemed one of hapless distortion and disintegrity. Often destructive to vulnerable others, including clients, their hapless projections somehow at the end of the day were to be forgiven.

The very empowerment they had garnered from mindbody work which they did imaginatively and responsibly, at some critical point seemed to sanction their acting out. In each lineage I examined, I felt confounded that the so-called practitioner-experts perpetrated the very patterns in which they were so-called removal experts, often simultaneously. And I could see myself doing the same. Why was I expecting more from them than this?

After the dry toast of psychoanalysis, I feasted on the juicy, adventuresome spirit of Moreno, the developer of psychodrama, and the neo-Reichians (Sharaf, Pierrakos, Lowen, Dillinger, and others), whose remarkable, brilliant, and often honest work I watched and experienced. Yet, father's son that I was, I sensed some personal compromise in their approaches.

They touched, but often for me at critical points they did not connect in a sustained, boundaried intimacy with the client's body. As practitioner, I needed more profound direct touch and holding than was their rule. I was looking for an entry point but found myself not wanting to apprentice in the ways which were offered.

And when push came to sometimes literal shove, these mindbody practitioners often retreated to analytic strategies to get their bearings. As theorists, the neo-Reichians were trying to get out from under the shadow of Reich's catastrophic demise at the hands of Freudian paranoia, establishment authoritarianism, and governmental concern about fringe energetic theory in the 1950s.

Perhaps identifying with the aggressors, some second generation Reichians put on the cloak of authority, becoming restrictive in the transmission of their lineage, for a time limiting training only to carefully selected doctors, as had Reich, with some exceptions. Certainly the trauma of governmental abuse of Reich, as well as Reich's own lineage, must have helped lead them in that direction.

But with clients, and sometimes therapists who were not afraid in workshops to become client, stripped down to their underwear, they sought to make honest, fearless, direct connection, pounding pillows, kicking, shouting, holding, and crying. Gratefully I was and still am deeply moved by their vision of connection I previously had thought impossible.

I realized for myself that I needed to go with greater specificity into what Reich calls our *character armor*, the embodied rigidities which I had felt psychologically, emotionally, and ultimately physically as I interacted with other people. Dismayed by the verbal and emotional hiatus that psychotherapy had evoked in me and others, I aligned myself with a like-minded lineage of Rolfing, which then held little truck with psychology. Our patterning was located in the structure of our bodies, and if we did not get that balanced and moving in relationship to gravity, nothing else would move.

I began my apprenticeship in touching bodies, practicing bodywork, and by the early 1980s, I was certified as a Rolfer, with the espoused intention of literally getting my hands upon the armor. With perhaps some fundamentalist intuition, I hoped I could realign, push, hold, and melt down these patterns, providing agency wherein I could participate and witness transformation. The resultant clear interaction would take place right under my fingers, without denial, without words or ideas, a place where the bull could not wriggle away, or fall asleep.

The therapeutic encounters I experienced and witnessed at workshops were blends of cognitive, emotional, and physical personal declaration, as therapists and clients imaginatively sought to bring mind and body together. Meditational modalities and martial arts were also offering avenues to wholeness. During this time, I began to have experiences witnessing so-called subtle energy as energy, rather than as character, character armor, or physiological structure.

The Energetic

After my experience with tragedy and Jane Austen, and the energetic stasis of psychoanalysis, my second direct experience with the body energetic occurred under the hands of George Dillinger, a California bioenergetic and gestalt therapist. I lay down on a mattressed surface and held my legs in the air for about ten minutes, while George placed his hands upon my belly and chest in various sequences.

Within a few minutes, I was aware of an increased sense of non-orgasmic pulsating, vibrating in a way I had never experienced. Waves of cellular tingling coursed throughout my body, including my face and mouth, which became distorted by the flow. My eyes seemed to radiate energy and to receive radiation from the light surrounding me. In Reichian terms, I thought I was "streaming."

I felt an urge to move as a way to manage the sensations, and I experienced an interface between the flow of energy and subsequent movement. After twenty minutes experiencing this flow, I perceived my defenses slowly rolling back into my system again, like tectonic plates resealing along the hull of my mindbody. When I asked George what it was all about, he wisely said, "I don't know."

" What can I do with this knowledge?" I asked him.

" I don't know," he again replied.

My third direct experience with the energetic (I did not call it that then, and do so now with some reservations) occurred with a diagnosis of a duodenal ulcer, which blossomed while on a vacation with my parents-in-law, during which every evening I drank a cocktail. The pain of the ulcer was new to me, and it was assuaged only by antacid pills. Within a week, I was placed on an antacid and custard diet which was supposed to continue indefinitely until I healed.

I began reflexology treatments, which were the only thing that gave relief from the pain in my gut. Hating the antacid diet, I began working with Rosemary Keene, a massage therapist who was acquiring bioenergetic techniques. Thus within a matter of months, I moved from psychoanalysis, flat on my back, fully clothed, to standing stark naked pounding pillows, shouting and bending backwards over high stools in order to increase my systemic tension prior to collapse.

I had started my work with Rosemary as a massage client, and I would flinch whenever she started to touch me. She noted that she had never seen someone in such pain. With exercises and practice, I gradually learned how to express the pain I had been only peripherally aware of.

Because the bioenergetic pounding of pillows had segued directly from the massage work, I kept my clothes off for the bioenergetic sessions. For these I could not later claim modesty because I had begun them nude. Exhilarated by the freedom, and politely ignoring any needs for ordinary decorum, it took me a year finally to put my exercise shorts back on.

For that year, I hunted amid interior landscapes, trying to connect with the pain I was manifesting to others. I learned how to breathe into pain, even when I was not sure where it was. On my return to Florida the next year, the ulcer acted up again. Foolishly I was sipping bourbon as I watched the evening sunsets.

My Ulcer Heals

One morning there I felt the ulcer pain in my left side come back, only this time, in a focusing moment, I breathed into it. Suddenly I was jolted by some connection heretofore not made, and some, for lack of a better term, energy thrust from the apparent site of my ulcer pain up into and out my eyes, with an electric force as if I had stuck my finger in a light socket.

The power of the connection was such that I dropped onto my adjacent bed and simultaneously sensed I would never be bothered by the ulcer again. I knew some major chemical, structural shift had occurred. After subsequent days of residual healing, I have not been bothered by the ulcer since.

I had read psychoanalytic literature claiming that an ulcer was a pre-verbal response to the absences of the mother, which the infant elaborates with energetic conviction in the following way:

1. If the food is not here when I want it, my mother is starving me. When it is obvious she returns late, but with food, she is still a bad mother, because my memory is now that she is someone who disappoints. So,

2. She is not starving me, rather she is poisoning me, as in Snow White and the poison apple. The infant fixes the site of the imagined poison energetically along the lining of its stomach, which becomes a tissue weakness which blossoms into an ulcer some twenty years later, as in my case.

After my jolting experience, I read Bergler, another analytic theorist specializing in what he called psychic masochism. He wrote that such ulcer "implantation" did not occur at Freud's oral stage, as one might suppose, but was developmentally prior to it at a visual stage, when the infant begins to see or not see the mother coming with the food. In fact, the energetic, electromagnetic connection of my ulcer pain with its pointed expression out my eyes, suggested a truth to this strategy.

More significantly, I saw that all the convolutions of psychoanalytic jargon and writing at best were describing the energy, not the ideation, of our psyches. I began to witness ideas as something different from what I thought them to be, perhaps as much reflections or reports about chemistries as about the structures or approaches to external reality.

When I discussed these insights with an analyst acquaintance of mine, known for his defensive arrogance, he flatly claimed there was no such ulcer literature in the analytic tradition. He opposed what I told him about my self-healing at every point, and finally begrudgingly offered, "Well, I guess you are left with your own experience," as if that were the most degrading option I could endure.

His response was not universal among therapists with whom I discussed my ulcer process, but the lack of respect for what is not understood made it difficult for me to comprehend the people who did not respect me or my experience. Some had significant difficulty with my story and tried to reframe it within their pseudo-rational professional rubrics.

I felt the separation between what I had experienced and knew and what for some psychology and psychiatry professionals was sadly beyond their capacity to relate to. The receptive ones were playful with my ideas and exploration, congratulating me and sharing their own stories of self-healing.

This cure revealed to me healing forces within myself which could be activated by myself by a curious kind of letting go, something I had not quite ever believed, nor been led to expect as possible by any regular physicians. Later, I used acupuncture, which addressed the *chi* energies, preventively facilitating the energetic, metabolic connections with needles and heat. I also felt the increasing primacy of the energy as opposed to ideation, which for me apparently had been the beacon toward which I steered my ship.

Tiffen and Former Lives

A fourth venture into the energetic came from ideation, and its occurrence had a typically Zen configuration. A friend suggested I get a former-life reading from Gregge Tiffen, who was visiting Boston, where I lived. The cost was $50 for ten minutes, and we could bring a tape recording with us, so that we did not have to forget a single, expensive moment.

Gregge was following the then-chic strategy of changing his name spelling as a way of taking on the responsibility for his own birth and naming. The night before the session, he gave a public briefing wherein he answered questions and talked a bit about what he was and was not going to do. He appeared with his silver-gray hair coiffed, wearing a golden cashmere jacket and white silk turtleneck with a medallion around his neck. He could not have seemed to me more plastic, and to someone raised in the conservative, up-tight East Coast, his deep, throaty resonances were equally untrustworthy.

I raised an existential question about where he felt he got his authority for this work, which he did not answer particularly to my satisfaction, and I began to sense a scam. Having signed up, however, I felt I would pay my money and at least have a story to tell.

In my session with him, Gregge quickly told me that I had had a bad death in the Charge of the Light Brigade, and that as a middle-rank officer I distrusted authority because I realized my men and I were being slaughtered in the exalted name of the English monarchy, but that there was actually no glory in such dying. Far from it, I had died in the awareness of radical, squalid betrayal by an authority I had believed in, an experience that had challenged belief itself. After a few more minutes of this, I paid Gregge my $50, took my tape and left.

What I did with this "information," however, was different from what heretofore I had done examining ideas. In the lineage of intellectual historians and of writers such as George Poulet, I had trained myself to enter belief systems as a believer, assuming that, if I did not approach the system from within, I could never find the fulcrum or initiating point of the system. Intuitively, I wanted to discover the center or point of present time out from which the writer was emotionally, psychodynamically writing what s/he was writing.

Rather than reason about the viability of former lives or not, or whether I should believe in such a construct, I simply took the idea in, this time watching what the experience of being told a former life did to me energetically in my mindbody. What I discovered was that, right away, some very deep holding pattern was touched. A level of anxiety seemed lessened by Tiffen's intervention as I felt a weight was lifting at a level I could sense but could not rationalize.

I had been raised within a Protestant, liberal arts, acculturated lineage where issues of faith were held at arms length: What could not dovetail with a kind of Presbyterian determinist rationality was better left alone, or approached cautiously. Yet the proposal of a former life placed my awareness in a new register where I had to revaluate my understanding of history, both as I knew it, and as I experienced it within myself.

The Pebble Drops into My Pond

Over time, this pebble's drop into my pond radiated in inexplicable and increasingly profound ways, as I allowed the idea to percolate within me. What I sensed was that the question became not whether reincarnation was true or not, or whether I believed it or not, but what it did to and within my systems as I knew them.

I had rejected life-after-death constructs as cruelly projective and filled with fantasy. When it came down to it, probably I was existentially stoic. This life is bounded permanently by our birth and our death, with no spill-overs. My mother's rational, internalized voice warned me that reincarnation is a defense against the difficulty of death, an escape for those who could not handle death's finality.

I had found her strategy true and good, and one I did not want to give up, yet I also saw a truth of reincarnation within myself. I had to admit that I could not honestly say what happens beyond death, but I began to see that such soul recycling added playful resonances against a hard core determinism which was influencing and limiting my current attitudes toward myself. What I saw with the narrative Gregge had given was the exposure of some organismic, cellular anxiety about dying—now I had been told that I had already died more than once and presumably could do it again. That was a very different way of confronting my death.

Using this construct as a mythic, spiritual flashlight, I could begin to face my death with some sense of playfulness, rather than as I had before, with some curious kind of perhaps disembodied rationality. Whether reincarnation was true or not again was not the issue. My perhaps stress about death and my difficulty in finding a way to approach death beyond the existential spiritualism that was as close as I could get to a viable belief was diminishing. The former-life strategy took me directly to my death in a manageable way.

I was evaluating this idea system by its effect upon my neurochemistry, not upon my reason, nor faith. Thus I discovered I was able to be more present within the complexities of the layering of identities which reincarnation suggested as I met with people and addressed myself. Rather than an escape, reincarnation could be an avenue to increased depth of exchange and self-awareness.

The 1960s and 1970s brought forward this mythology with a vengeance, and I ran into people who used reincarnation to aggrandize, to grandiose, or to fundamentalize. They would become militant when I suggested that reincarnation was a strategy toward something else. They wanted to possess their former lives as actually lived, rather than hover with these narratives at some other level.

I had seen how Tiffen had taken some reading of me, including my question at the briefing and had referred it back to me, not in an analytic, distancing way, but in a narrative which invited my involvement with my issues in a form I could appropriate and study. But even such narrative was not the bottom line.

The genius of the strategy became increasingly pronounced as I approached people as fellow migrant souls, densifying, incarnating within bodies, bringing with them patterns for resolution which began outside our current time frame, but which could be resolved within these four dimensions in our here and now. Rather than dwelling in some former-life fantasy, reincarnation made clear to me that no matter what our former lives, in this lifetime we are who we are, not who we have been.

To Learn

Most significantly in this regard, as Tiffen pointed out, I saw our essential task here on earth is to learn, to learn about the patterns, transmitted from the past, and to let them go in order to be, not just to become. So many of the struggles and achievements of the American sixties and seventies rocketed between the axis of becoming and being, and reincarnation as a strategy focuses with consistency upon that fulcrum.

I could not give up my Protestant intellectualism, passed through to me primarily from my parents. Nor could I deny the possibility of reincarnation, which held equal power. Both strategies were true, and both of them commented upon death. I would have to embrace a dual reality and somehow pass into seeing both contradictory systems as avenues to some mystery which narrative itself belied. As with the analytic jargon about ulcers, I saw that what ideas are true about is not ideas, nor their juxtaposition, nor so-called rationality, but about dropping into a level of mystery beyond narrative.

I became adept at intuiting the patterns I saw, the sufferings of others which were otherwise nameless, and by giving them narrative form, making them user-friendly. I could say things which allowed shifts in judgment and potentialities approximating humor, and this playfulness became a hallmark of my understanding about the nature of human reality. I could be both light and deep, rather than just heavy and deep, as often I had a reputation for being.

The ultimate proof of reincarnation was in the pudding, in my ability to use the strategy with grace and humor, not with rigidity. Likewise I could not clutch at my belief that there was no life after death as the existentialist 1940s and 1950s had encouraged me to proclaim. That strategy was itself an achievement born out of the moral chaos engendered under Christian after-life mythology. I was confronting not life after death, which had a curious, linear sense of present tense, but lives after deaths, a very different chemistry and one that challenged my old sense of history.

The ideas and belief systems were not to be held tightly, or the mystery could not be witnessed. I had known this intellectually, because I had trained to enter and drop out of such systems with alacrity; that was a sign of intelligence, and a primitive preamble to wisdom. Now I began to acknowledge at a deeper level that belief was not where I wanted to be, but rather that *being* meant knowledge, of a new, initially paradoxical sort.

The points of entry and exit to this human existence as parts of the continuum of my life were challenged, and with those challenges I saw the limits of my understanding of time and specifically the encapsulations of my understanding of history, personal and public. At death, time disappears, or changes, or is different beyond our understanding, and all after-life considerations are projections of what we know or don't know here and now. Using this approach, I could begin to find out what it is I can know.

A child of a culture with a linear cosmology about Heaven and Hell, which was not encouraged within my family, I could bounce now between existential austerity and reincarnation and land in some realm within myself which was true and beyond ordinary narrative, cognition, and sensation. This was beyond the world of recordable energy, approaching through its subtle periphery, my experience of Spirit.

I thanked unbelievable Tiffen for transmitting to me in his almost rejectable mannerism, an age-old lineage. I continue to feel it has been the best single $50 I have spent. I found myself assembling experiences that embraced both the energetic and my overtly physical incarnation, particularly the structural focus of hands-on bodywork and Rolfing.

Rolf and Connective Tissue

Ida Rolf, the developer of structural integration or Rolfing, focused her search for the locus of the point of origin of held patterning at the level of *connective tissue* and its chemistry. Rolf had studied chiropractic, with its focus upon spine alignment, and yoga, and she knew about approaching stress reduction by paying attention to muscles and their attachments. As a biochemist, she intuited that the shortcomings and often temporary fix-it results of these approaches could be obviated by addressing a different level of organization in the body structure, namely the connective tissue.

In one of a series of Rolfing sessions, wearing only underwear, the client (Rolfee) lies upon a low, knee-high table while the Rolfer renders a deep, structurally intentioned pressure and manipulating "massage," using hands and arms upon the client's body surfaces. Gradually, as connective tissue is revitalized, bone, muscle, and proprioceptive awareness of the body alter, resulting in greater ease of movement and reduction of stress.

Rolf proposed that trauma introduces distortions in this system of connection and communication with all parts of the body. By means of locating and bringing client brain to focus upon these holding places, often to the point of deep sensation, including initially pain, our entire human structure could be released and educated into new levels of integrity, in relationship to gravity, now experienced as a support, not a drag.

Rolf saw how energy applied at this level by an exterior source, the Rolfer, could radically transform many human structures, externally visible and interiorly sensible. This it appeared to do, but not all the time, and not predictably. Huge changes occurred in some people, and yet some patterning was not affected. Critically, in many Rolfers who embodied the lineage, amid the balance of our bodies there remained immaturities, both physical and emotional.

Seeing this, I returned to my drawing board, not rejecting the Rolfing, which I feel can hold many important pieces in the healing puzzle. My intuition about why Rolf chose the "incarnate" level of connective tissue collagen and the wrappings which encompass and link all parts of the body is that, like those in spiritual traditions, she was seeking the surest point of reference from which to purview our entire mindbody experience.

Structural integration would also be the most efficient, least complex approach toward transformation, because the connective tissue is where the body's structural "compass" is located and neurophysiologically set. From this point of view, I saw connective tissue, itself a communication system, as the physical location equivalent of ego, of psychological integrity, the physiological place-grid which connects all the parts of the body together. I later intuited that from an energetic point of view, the connective tissue was Rolf's appropriate focus, because that was where it was safest for Rolf to approach her own traumata.

The fact that she allowed her lineage to be transmitted intrusively and abusively suggests that her point of entry, at the level of connective tissue holding, may have been a "rescue station" from a deeper immobility surrounding abuses which she could only partially, perhaps never, approach. Distressed by the ineffectuality of psychodynamic therapeutic excesses, many early Rolfers, including Rolf, chose only to rotate their clients' tires and change their oil, rather than discuss feelings with them.

That imbalance in the teaching lineage has since been redressed, and the style, while still deep, in the second and third generations of teachers and students, has been rendered more responsive to the client's whole process. Yet in her recipe, Rolf revolutionized the conduct of bodywork for clients and practitioners, expanding the intellectual, physical, sensate, and imaginative limits of what could be sought and delivered on the table.

Until the late 1980s, I continued as a Rolfer, functioning at the humanistic, psychodynamic end of the Rolfing continuum. I then expanded and overtly focused my practice to include victims of sexual and physical abuse. In this I encountered some success based upon a level of equality and respectful attention to the complete client process, psychodynamic as well as structural, which I sought to bring to the Rolfing situation. I was still attached to words and psychodynamic issues, though often my Rolfing sessions were conducted in relative silence.

There were some notable successes based upon a reciprocity of experience between me and the Rolfee and the trust that engendered. There were also clients who were beyond my skill to help. They reacted to my offering of trust, and even playfulness, with rejection and fear which I found discouraging and at times almost inexplicable, though characteristically I questioned my own approaches.

A fifth main experience with the energetic occurred in the 1980's, when, through my wife's connection with her, I began listening to Vimala Thakar, a practitioner of awareness meditation, and a friend of Krishnamurti, whom I had studied when in graduate school. Her continued articulate focus upon the holistic, energetic truth and the curse of fragmentation by ego which keeps us from embodying that confirmed and deepened my awareness of the importance of moving beyond words and thought constructs into the silence of the energetic.

It is she who greets her listeners, not as followers of a guru or even students of a teacher, but as friends, fellow inquirers into the nature of reality and awareness in relationship with her. In her life, she has eschewed organizations, power, the trappings of success, speaking and writing only to those who request it. The influence of her presence and clarity as a support to my life continues to expand into the present. As much as any, she has provided a model of integrity based upon my understanding of energy and the clear.

With Levine

Listening in 1993 to Levine and his few, telling examples drawn not from tragedy and tragic theory, but from scientific literature about animals and trauma, brought all of the earlier classical material back: My preoccupations with tragic immobility (*stasis*), recognition (*anagnōrisis*), change (*metabasis*), pride (*hubris*), reversal (*peripeteia*), etc.

More critically, I focused upon how my understanding of the life force and of subtle energies fit into Levine's retrospective upon what scientific and social science people had been evolving in the understanding of trauma over the past one hundred years. For me it dovetailed with a lineage of concern that had been addressed humanistically for over 2,500-5,000 years, and my inner sight was expanded and confirmed by Levine's presentation and with the work I had done with him on my own at least forty-six year-old trauma pattern.

CHAPTER TWO:
TRAUMA AND HELD ENERGY

The Trauma Mechanism

In the expansion of energy released by my work on trauma after encountering Levine in Boulder, including my accident stepping on the glass, I saw things monolithically, messianically, to put it mildly and accurately. In the first flush of a new level of insight, my mind integrated, organized around the following perspective. Here, composed on the airplane returning to Boston, with Reichian, oracular conversion fervor, is what I wrote:

"There is only one function in the mindbody which must be mastered, and that is the mechanism of trauma. All stress and disease which we currently label as such are derived from this mechanism. It is the "reason" for divorce, for conflict, for the ups and downs of the stock market, for in fact all aspects of what we think of as culture and all attempts to correct culture's problems. It is the fountainhead of lineages of abuse, perpetrated overtly and covertly by humankind. It is the source of all suffering, and the misunderstanding of this mechanism is the source of all suffering and sin.

"Understanding trauma provides the corrective answer to the questions of racism, totalitarianism, all fundamentalist ideations with their resultant conflicts and scourges, of violence, of history, to psychological and physiological crippling; and, by tracing and releasing traumatic holding, we can envision the promise of ecstatic, transcendent living. Comprehension of its power, and the simple ways it operates, may yield a conclusion to cancers, immuno-deficiency syndromes, and the like, not to mention our concern with the common cold. Within its features lies the end of war and our resistance to peace.

"In the history of the world, major idea systems have assisted human transformation by approaching in some perhaps partial, perhaps in rare cases completing way the territory I now see as the trauma mechanism.

"All of the horrors of the past one hundred centuries and of the twenty-first to come are derived from an empatterned execution of the traumatic mechanism within the individual and the society within which that individual lives. It is the extension of this pattern which has resulted or perhaps will result in the end of the habitable world.

"Hence the first objective of all education should be the training of young people to recognize and cease the perpetuation of abusive patterns visited upon them by the agency of this mechanism by adults and fellow children. We are bullied, and in the attempt to rid ourselves of that pattern, we seek out situations which duplicate the initial trauma memory of that bullying, and so we bully; but we start as receptors of traumatic impact. The trauma of our Civil War, with its roots in European entitlement, is projected upon the civil war of Vietnam, where it seeks "safe" completion beyond our American soil.

"From this viewpoint, crucially, perpetrator and victim are seen as victims alike, for victims within the agency of trauma perpetrate its patterns upon themselves and often upon others until the patterns are dissolved.

Initial Guidelines

"What are the hallmarks of the trauma mechanism, and how can their simplicity be gleaned from the wealth of apparently varied experience which it generates? A few initial guidelines are listed here.

"We can choose to address problems from many positions in our neurochemistry. But at some point, we have to give up the idea that we can maintain a fixed perspective. Since internal landscapes are too varied, we have to achieve a more flexible understanding. Ideas in their rigidities juxtapose with such apparent painful contradictory force that we have to seek more general, fluid, high ground from which to establish an apparently consistent overview of what we are experiencing.

"Christians and Jews achieve this high ground with the experience of the Holy Spirit; easterns by the chi, prana, and kundalini; Freudians by libido, etc. All these strategies complete the questions:

" 'What is universal and constant which will transcend the vicissitudes of ideational and emotional change within our human experience?'

" 'Can this "position" provide a stable point from which to view the vagaries of experience?'

" 'Where, or better, from what marker, can we best find, identify and witness the underlying organization of experience? Can we find a true point of origin for our being, and is that the best place to view our experience overall? And is that location what we mean by soul?'

"To ground our intellectual functioning and to stabilize it, we turn to the sense of flow within ourselves, our experiencing of the neurochemistry of twitching, pulsating, of sexuality, meditation, breathing, and digesting, of moving. We then ask how we are experiencing that energy, which may be characterized as metabolic, chemical, and spiritual.

"Following Nietzsche's lead, Shaw called our life energy the *life force*, which is a perspective from which one can observe the power of movement in character, physical activity, and even social interactions. Bergson called the life force *elan vitale*, Hahnemann called it the *vital force*, the Reiki art of healing identifies it as the universal life force; it is also the focus of the Tao. We can all disagree about the varied details by which we can know it.

"What people in disagreement have been doing over many generations is to challenge the perspective of the viewer, based upon what he is reporting. 'You are not looking at the life force from the appropriate viewpoint,' they argue, 'hence what you say about it is biased and ultimately limited.' Are these real grounds for disagreement or agreement? And do they in any significant way matter?

Agreement

"As in the film-story of *Rashomon*, we have been a bit like various witnesses to an assault, seeing aspects of a truth, yet a truth which is verbally expressed and perceived through the authority of the thought and verbal centers of the brain. Often in the history of disagreements, what appeared to be threatened by challenging ideas was the hierarchical authority of the thought centers of the brain, not the ideas which they supposedly issue and trade. Our life energy can describe itself, but there is a risk to that task, both for the agency describing and the energy described.

"From whichever attitudinal 'places' our life energy is viewed, those places generate our differences and our agreements. Why are we so preoccupied with differences when we are talking about the same reality? We continue to have serious conflicts arising because of disagreements about reality.

"For example, if we were to say to people who disagree about the nature of God, 'The basic premise about that which you both are arguing is the same, for you and the other whose views you now challenge. Your task now is to present your differences while acknowledging that you are speaking about the same thing,' what would be the nature of their ensuing discussion? Would we, or they, consider it a disagreement, or a discussion, or what? What if the argument entailed the participants asking each other, 'Why are you using different words to describe the same thing I am?'

"For real estate, the three most important things determining the value of a property are location, location, and location. In the same way, it seems to me that the crippling limitation of perspective is what all the fighting has been about. The history of ideas reveals variations of approaches to the same unitary, elusive phenomenon, the trauma mechanism and its relationship to life energy. Life energy is whole. In thought and in trauma we experience division. In irrational disagreement, we experience the cost of traumatic splitting.

"We can drop into any time and place to find commentary and attempts to scale its problematic walls, and to reduce its toxicity. From Buddha's teachings to Jesus' parables, to Groddeck's *It*, the goal is reclaiming the life force which somehow gets stilled. Like the common cold, everyone has a cure, yet colds continue to occur, and people elaborate upon their occurrence."

Well, that was what poured out. I hope you can sense the intensity which this focus engendered. Involved with the life force, spirit tradition in the humanities, as I returned to Boston, I was determined to explore this insight perspective. And I was again thrown upon my own devices.

In his teaching, Peter focused on the neuromechanics of trauma, as well as the emotional and cognitive aspects of symbolic apperception of patterning. He did not then characterize or acknowledge the life force vector as erotic, as I, immersed in the Freud-Reich lineage, intuited it was. In variance from that lineage, however, I intuited that the energy was not necessarily orgasmically sexual. Among other matters, I wondered what that awareness might do to his consideration of the underlying energetics of sexual abuse trauma.

Sexual Abuse

In my work with victims of sexual abuse, I had sensed that the problem might not lie so much in the facts of the abuse, though these can be enormously difficult, but rather in the cognitive perception and storage of those facts which the victims found most disturbing. The victims I saw had done everything they could to recover *the* critical memories, but they remained helpless to change the patterns that tormented and disrupted their lives.

Erica, a twenty-nine year-old ballerina recovering from a severe ankle injury, came initially to me for Rolfing. She complained as well of a chronic twist in her neck. Facing the abrupt end of her career in dance, she noted wryly, "I could have been a contender."

Over time, her story emerged. At the age of two, her father died and her mother remarried. She adored her stepfather and would give him backrubs. One night while rubbing his back when she was four, the stepfather rolled over in bed revealing an erection.

Innocently loving the man, Erica started to fellate him, yet as the man began to have an orgasm, he held the girl's head down on his penis, choking her. The girl tried to kick away, but was momentarily impaled. A confusing interface of erotic, sexual, and life-threatening forces was set in place in the four year-old's neurochemistry.

Erica continued to have sexual experiences with her stepfather until she was eleven, when she left her dysfunctional home, where she had taken care of her brothers and avoided the toxicities of her mother's alcoholism. She reported that, as an adult, she did not hold particular anger toward her stepfather for breaching her trust. As a young woman, she tried heterosexual marriage, as well as lesbian relationships, but neither adjustment worked out. She could not make either lifestyle fit and was always on the outside.

Charming and in many ways remarkably balanced, at twenty-seven, a week after another surrogate father died ("the only *father* I really knew"), as she was dancing particularly well one night, Erica's heel caught in the hem of a special costume, and she smashed her ankle, virtually destroying her premiere ballerina's career.

What Erica and I came to wonder was whether the brain, in its moment of high vibrationality, brings forward a traumatic pattern, in this case, the life and death struggle of the loving, confounded, suffocating girl. She began the erotic experience with tenderness and love, but at a certain point, the stepfather's sexuality apparently becomes adult and objectified. He objectifies the girl, turning her into a body that performs in a terrifying, confusing series of moves in which the child cannot get enough air.

Erica later became a performer in the dance, and twenty-three years after, at the peak of her career, in the full vibrational trust which grief can entail, we strategized that brain addresses the trauma, probably twisting the head and kicking away. Brain attempts to cast off the role of objectified performer which had been traumatically laid in as a four year-old whose eros had been traumatized, we might say betrayed.

In other ways after her accident, Erica later demonstrated her reluctance to "perform" without adequate preparation. What seemed interesting to us both was how her erotic, joyful, innocent reaching out, her loving, might have been turned by the step-parent into a *held-energy system* which sought completion for many years, and finally, radically discharged, at significant cost to the victim. Thus what Erica and I proposed was her recovery of the unalloyed erotic life force in that portion of her neurochemistry where it was being held.

Erica moved to the West Coast, and we still work together when she returns for visits. She continues the slow process of recovery, finding movement where before there was stasis.

A New Approach

Supported by my new and revived insights and focus as a result of my time in Boulder, I began working directly with traumatic patterning with those of my Rolfing clients who were interested. Instead of stripping down to their underwear as they do for a Rolfing session, clients remained clothed on the table, facing the ceiling. Intuitively, I began to hold them at the neck and base of the spine.

For over six months, I sat at one side of the table or the other, holding my hands in this fashion without moving them for up to ninety minutes per session, until it affected my shoulder girdle and wrists. I decided to move up to the head end of the table and to sit holding the client at the base of the neck using two hands.

I asked them not to move too much in order to allow the energy to complete the pattern by itself. To keep them comfortable, I placed a pillow under their knees and legs. Seated and resting my arms on my knees, I could make this latter solution less taxing for me, and intuitively it seemed to offer a better energetic balance, conveying a sense of support and connection.

Elise

As many mindbody practitioners do, I encouraged clients to focus upon their inner experience in the present situation. "Where is the twitch?" "Where does it hurt?" "Can you describe the pain in greater detail?" "What seems to be happening here?" "How old are you in this memory?" and "Who is there with you?" were the sort of orienting questions I would ask. We quickly found not only sensations, but stories and insights.

Elise, a body therapist, is arching her head to the right as she lies on the table. "What is happening?" I ask her.

"I am seven, and I am being beaten by my father. He's drunk."

"Why is he beating you?" I ask.

"Actually, he is beating my mother, because she won't perform sexually for him," she explains. "I stand between them to protect my mother. After a while I get frustrated with the impasse, and I say, 'OK, Dad, I'll do it for you'." And she services him sexually until she is fourteen.

I come to understand this as a narrative paradigm of the way in which eros in the child, our outward-reaching life energy, gets transmuted in a protective, compassionate way, informing the distortions of the interactions between abusing parent and child. What Elise acts out is what I think as infant energy systems we all do with the parental patterns we confront. Like any universal so-called Christ child, we take on the "sins" of our world out of compassion, before we can know their long-term, crippling impact upon us. And in the process we become traumatized and co-dependent.

As infants, we respond to our surround in full trust, and what our parent's brain gives back is its traumatic pattern, probably gained from its parents. The lineage is either transmitted through activity, or indirectly through feelings and attitudes or directly at an energetic level. Even amid the majestic, swirling, foetal symphony of the womb, the information is all conveyed perhaps for generations without interruption or awareness.

The earliest disconnections from the life force may be declared where love cannot be felt by young children. There are questions whether this truncation is a function of traumatic patterning, or of just having to learn how to love from reconstituted, revisory parenting. My own preference with clients is to discover how the inherent life force may be erotic and compassionate even at conception, with later infringements traumatically imposed. This strategy suggests an almost universal application of this understanding of trauma process at every level, a simplification, to be sure, but one which may lead directly to held-energy systems and their resolution.

Moreover, I intuited that the trauma mechanism itself, producing held-energy systems, causes the deepest trouble for our brains. These systems' apparently idiosyncratic pattern of self-concealment and disclosure cannot be fathomed at ordinary levels. I think this is what causes so much distress and suffering, and draws such fire when mirrored in an external social milieu where perpetrators deny what they have done. Or victims are blamed.

One summary insight I came to was that our traumata are omnipresent, always waiting in the wings to take stage center and to complete, *this* time successfully. This condition is true for me and for everyone I meet—can there be exceptions? This means that I do not face people, but patterns (was I prepared to call them masks?), imitations of serious action, *dramatis personae* whose characteristics are determined by traumatic structures. Aristotle's mimesis becomes a sure signal of the presence of dissociative traumatic processing, essential to tragic configuring.

These characteristics appear to us, their caretakers, stable to the point of rigidity. In illusion we believe them stable until we see how they are laid in and how they can be allowed to leave. These densities may express the lineages of trauma conveyed through family and cultural lines going back hundreds of years; and they appear right on the edge of resolution in every moment. Only with those who are *clear* is there a possibility of real dialogue free of encapsulation shadowing.

Suddenly the uniformity of this vision itself became more recognizable to me, and the world shrank in interrelational complexity. My task seemed simple enough. I could not go back to study more science and meaning and symbol, all of which appeared to lead in the direction of retraumatization of the energy. Like Diogenes, I had to follow my own direction, and, lamp aloft, search for wholeness, my own honesty.

Watch Brain Do the Work

In my practice, as we witnessed what the client mindbody was revealing in the current present as client lay sensating on the table, it became increasingly certain that, if observant, and lucky, client and I could watch the trauma completion take place. Sometimes clients would be emotionally moved by the vividness that was evoked, and they would cry, or struggle to find some release.

Yet the more I worked with clients at this level, the more I came to distrust a superficial release, emotional or physical. My intuition was that these therapeutic releases illuminate if you have never experienced them, but often they do not take the pattern out. So I cautioned clients not to spend a great deal of time in emotion, or movement, as we had been trained to do by therapists since Freud.

Increasingly I asked them to remain still, to watch *brain* do the work. This work was not physical, or "emotional," or a function of will or intention. It engaged that which organized the emotional and physical, namely the energy level which *incarnated* into the experience we call *mindbody*, where what we think of as *mind* meets and interconnects with what we think of as *body*.

I use the term incarnation here somewhat technically to indicate the process whereby spirit becomes densified into energy and into mindbody. And increasingly I came to use the word *brain* to help *mind*, the energetic of the body which we think of as ourselves, to reconnect with its incarnate physical location, our neurochemistry in our nervous system. That mind then passes through a fundamentalist view of body to a renewed perception of its essence as energy can be seen as the main business of trauma resolution.

Where many in the psychotherapeutic lineages were proposing gently entering the trauma memory by therapeutic focus upon a system of meaning and symbols and gradual, trusting accommodation, I intuited a hopefully safe, simpler organization. Somewhat outside the Reichian lineage, Levine and others focus differently upon what is stilled by trauma process, stressing a locked fight-or-flight sequencing in the neurochemistry. I think they are wise in arguing for the restoration of that mechanism as a sign of full functioning to the individual.

Yet the relational, erotic vector of our life energy seemed to me also essential to witness as clients move into energetic levels beyond the narrative of fight or flight. I was increasingly captivated by the outward, flowing, holistic vibration of energy beyond the ordinary definitions of body boundaries at the skin, which was essential to my understanding, if only to know when mindbody balance is achieved.

For me, a more extensive recognition of the primacy of spiritual levels also seemed necessary, grounded as they were for me in Western traditions I had experienced in the religious and humanistic lineages of tragic theory. That was not what Levine and many classically trained clinicians were doing, nor trying to do, though like all healers, they were hanging out in the same territory.

Andrew

I continued with those Rolfees who wanted to experiment, sometimes in alternation with Rolfing sessions. With Rolfing, I had helped bring some relief to Andrew, a forty year-old migraine-plagued man who was at his wits' end. He had headaches stacked upon debilitating headaches and had been taking serious anti-headache medications for years with no conclusive success until, in one of our sessions, he located the point of origin of his pattern.

Scanning through his current mindbody experience while lying on the table, Andrew at one point noted, "This is where I start to have a five-day migraine." In spite of this risk, we agreed to venture forth. I asked him to identify the site of held energy by witnessing the colors, focusing particularly on black. I found myself encouraging him to divide the larger, impenetrable massing he saw into sub-particles.

Our sense was that brain was stymied at the size of the problem, so we chose to divide it into bite-sized portions, on the theory that the traumatized brain could extrapolate holographically and solve the entire system if it could neurochemically understand a representative part of it. At this new level, Andrew witnessed an energetic "particle" and noted his energy, something like his attention, going toward and away from the particle. After he delineated the shape he was watching, I asked, "What's its color?"

"Black," was his reply. With whatever faculty, through color and shape we sensed he could witness the eros of the life force moving toward and away from the held-energy problem, which was somehow familiar to him. Our fight-or-flight mechanism was in its essence relational and playful, not hostile and combative.

"How old is this pattern?" I asked.

"It's been there forever," he spoke with some despair.

"If it is forever, and not from a former life, could this pattern be prenatal?" I asked.

"I think so," he noted. "It feels terrible. It is driving me crazy."

Still focusing somewhat upon emotional and narrative strategies, I inquired, "If you are in the uterus, are you alone?"

"She's not there; my mother," he noted with some wonder.

"Can you sense where the mother is?" I asked. He became still and vigilant for a couple of moments.

"Oh," Andrew spoke quietly.

"Oh?"

"My mother," he slowly commented. "She's drinking. Not a lot. But it's too much." Then he added with some excitement, "It's shifting." After some more silences he reported witnessing the headache pattern leave from that configuration for the first time in his life. He was elated.

"Have we got some kind of fetal. . .alcohol something?" I asked playfully, fishing for categories I do not ordinarily use.

"I think maybe. I can't do anything with this particle, and it's toxic." After witnessing the mechanism, his mindbody became, for lack of a better term, preoccupied, slack, turning away.

"Are you discouraged?" I questioned. He nodded. "Why?" I asked.

"It's coming back," he noted. "The headache. I thought it was gone forever."

"Is it the same now as before?" I returned.

"No, it isn't; it isn't as intense," he admitted. Pausing, with greater spirit, he then added, "And I know how to get it out." We discussed various strategies, including flushing it out by drinking water, exhaling it, and the like. Now brain was engaged in the problem.

"How long will that take?" I asked.

"Six months," he intuited. He immediately felt a neurochemical shift toward optimism, and about six months later he reported he was off all medication with no significant headaches of the sort he had been experiencing all his life. "We broke the pattern's back," he reported three years later. After this session and others like it, I began to sense the possibility of profound, immediate self-healing connections with this technique.

I intuited that with the deepest trauma patterns, brain, not the dissociated energy we might call mind, must be allowed to do the work itself. The initial formulations of mind as self are dissociative, so both "client" and "practitioner" must get out of the way. I was providing a non-intrusive, non-intentional presence with my hands under Andrew's neck. It provided an energetic matrix which I thought served as a platform of relational trust. This trust activated the traumatic pattern surfacing for completion.

And I was strategizing with Andrew how to focus and observe, but essentially nothing more. We could reduce the narrative, the interpretation, the discussions drastically and focus upon what is essential. Where is brain stuck, and could mind, even dissociative awareness thought to be self, bring brain to that place in its chemistry? From this point of view, all remainders of technique seemed intervention. Where the pattern is most difficult, brain must figure it out, in the company of someone else, to provide a relational energy matrix, but not with interventional "help."

Doris

Doris, a therapist and a victim, is trying to solve the mystery of sexual abuse. She scans and finds her way into a black box which she discovers is hollow. We wonder about whose pattern that is, and she says, "It has something to do with the father." Its hollowness interests me. Perhaps, she and I consider, it is not the activities which are disturbing in her experience of sexual abuse.

Rather, perhaps, it is the child's experience of the hollowness of the activity, the energetic pressure of it which is traumatizing—its lack of reciprocity, and its developmentally premature rigidities. For most of us, our adult sexuality is urgent, filtering through the structures of our childhood trauma, and discharging, whether or not our pattern completes or transforms.

To impose this energetic upon a receptive child may reflect the desire to heal as well as the hapless retraumatization of the perpetrator, not to mention the inexplicable difficulty for a victim/child who also seeks to heal the parent in the mindbody of a child.

Now the memory of what "happened" to Doris is not certain, even when memory details are recalled. She and I muse together about reworking the pattern of hollowness which she is carrying. Her pattern becomes an energetic awareness, not a problem in unrecalled and unrecallable history.

She is not concerned with the familiar issue of responsibility and the victim/perpetrator axis which has gotten her nowhere. As child, she blames herself, as adult she blames the perpetrator; but that does not put the issue to rest. With excitement, we both see that such narrative analysis is secondary to getting the pattern out, which she intuits can be done, but not by narrative means.

Her brain is now interested in dissolving the pattern, which heretofore was considered impossible. She notes, "With the abuse, I lost my will, and do not know what help is. Help is not intervention." I find myself responding, "Help is allowing brain to move into the energetic. For the deepest patterns, no classical intervention will work. As minds, we can say, 'Brain must be allowed to solve it.'"

We meet occasionally over the next few months, and then she starts canceling, or missing appointments. A therapist herself, she does not respond to our mutually bemused, shared commentary about the reasons why she does not return. We continue to run into each other on the street, and we are still in that holding pattern, as far as I know.

History and Time

People are always rewriting history, but not in a way that is usually meant. To reclaim the traumatized energy is to move, and yet I think there is no history, no boat's wake, when we move with what is called *right action*. But history, as we have been trained the past is, appears based upon held-energy systems and our incomplete understanding of them.

In particular, within held-energy systems, there is no movement, hence no time. Here, as with right action, we are also out of ordinary, perhaps all time. Thus when we compose our histories, what we probably record is the history of traumatic understanding, of distortion memory. The consequences of not being able to change the patterns, not able to get to the fundamental positions where change occurs, are the residue that history describes.

My own understanding coalesced over the following months, with the following hallmarks. Trauma therapists seemed to be developing approaches featuring a multi-leveled system accounting for the variety of phenomena that trauma promulgates, including traditional psychological and medical diagnosis of symptom, as well as distortions in symbol, behavior, cognition, meaning, and the like. In contradistinction, my clients and I saw that these phenomena could be considered secondary, because the held energy which controls the point of origin of the stored trauma and the suffering is invisible to ordinary cognitive perception of the mind. We became even more direct.

I work with Harry, thirty-two, probably sexually abused as a boy by his father. On the table, he is arching his back in agony, silently struggling with some patterning he reports is the toughest thing in his life he has done. He seems to be at some confluence of memory and movement. I watch him move around some fixed point. I ask him, "Are you suffering?" He responds, "Yes."

I say, "Would you like to move out of suffering?" He nods. I say, "Focus on the black, as black, as if you are approaching the black portion of a picture, where you no longer recognize its shape, context, or meaning. Find the color and hang out there. See if that is the source of your suffering." He focuses upon the black.

"How does that feel?" Some deep tension pattern leaves him immediately. He says, "Something has changed." We both witness the alteration of something deep. It seems too simple, too easy. Yet something happens directly and indirectly which is rarely the rule in therapy or growth modalities.

In language we suffer; in thought we suffer; in reason and logic, in analysis, we suffer. In energy we ultimately solve, we move and become whole again.

We must begin in the place where there is no movement, no vibration, no color. I start to wonder whether those close to me who complain that they don't "get" my color technique are declaring part of the traumatic process. They cannot move into the energetic, or I cannot lead them there. They, and I with them, are with language, ego, and their decadent admixtures in which we hang out together and enjoy flashes of energy amid galaxies of held-energy systems. But we are not real, nor do we experience our wholeness.

Neurochemistries

At a new, deeper level than before, my clients and I reengage with the commonplace that we are *neurochemistries*. What we call our consciousness can be seen as a mere set of odd, strange corks floating on and within a chemical sea, transmitted by chemistries of communication throughout the neurons, neurotransmitters, endocrine, and tissue systems of the mindbody.

We can read in texts about neurochemistry, or we can take drugs, or food, or seek out experience to affect our moods which are altering our neurochemistries. But we seem to shy away from actually experiencing ourselves as people as neurochemistry. Unless we are in some allied scientific profession, we do not think, "Oh, this sadness is a neurochemistry," or "As I watch and experience my orgasm, I am watching and experiencing a neurochemistry, and that, from within, that neurochemistry is precisely what I am experiencing."

Educated in both the humanistic and later peripherally in some scientific disciplines, I found myself returning to the word *neurochemistry*, not from an exclusively scientific context, but blending the scientific usage with, say, a spiritual or humanistic one. And as I used it in commonplace language, to raise consciousness, my own, my friends', my clients', I found that I was also raising eyebrows, as if I had crossed some important and inviolable syntactical, rubric boundary.

Again, I posited that I could view my words, my thoughts, my subtle sense of myself as manifestations of something else, something prior and more important than the ideas, sensations, and feelings and thoughts. I, and my analyst, and all the therapists I had worked with had assumed these were primary, and, because of their often unique, sometimes recurring assembly, my own. All these phenomena, I now ventured, might be mimetic.

For me, my new usage invited participation of my awareness at the neurochemical level, rather than say, the psychodynamic one. It took me radically, quickly to the realm of the energetic, approximate, I felt, to what is called neurochemical and its point of origin.

What I seemed to be witnessing at some new energetic level was literally true, and literally was a neurochemistry, which in the other sense, is a commonplace insight. Or what I was witnessing was just prior to neurochemistry, which placed me at least in the realm of the energetic, next to and within spirit. I could have emotional responses, and active intellectual engagement with myself as a neurochemistry. As energetic, dissociated mind, I could reconnect with the primal energetic below traumatized physiology which I called brain.

I became more interested in observing the chemistry of my thoughts than in the ideas, feelings, and sensations which had seemed my essential reality. Increasingly, I saw these latter phenomena as mere *narrative*, imitating a serious action which could not be conventionally addressed but which is constantly being proposed as something in my mindbody and its agency, my brain chemistry and physiology.

Narrative, I proposed, is the label, the form, which is pasted on our energetic beings at the end of the assembly line of consciousness. Narrative includes our incarnation but is not the point of origin of the incarnation, at least not as perceived by most of us. Only when we are *clear* do we radiate our source through our narrative (*cf.* avatar traditions including Jesus, Gautama Buddha, Mohammed, the Lama and Zen traditions, etc.).

Fundamentalism

I was at a fulcrum of relationship between the movement of ideas and feelings, so-called experience, and something else. That something else was chemical, even atomic, and beyond or around that, energetic and spiritual. It could be directly apprehended, not as symbol, but as fact. I was not viewing imitation, but rather the serious action itself, between the narratives of energy and the mystery out of which they occur.

I felt myself peer over the edge of a guardrail into the very deep chasms of fundamentalism, yet I kept my bearings. I saw that the patterns of suffering could be met and transformed only if addressed and given sustained attention at this invisible, energetic level. It was not at verbal or physical levels which only expressed their form, but were not at the point of immobilization, the only important point of origin for suffering and her sister, change.

So my clients and I started to learn how to enter our energetic levels of awareness, and inspired by Levine's clarity, to which I added and modulated my own for me significant pieces of the puzzle, we fashioned an approach that would help people to focus upon this trauma mechanism, the very same territory I began to explore over thirty years before as a graduate student in England studying Aeschylus and tragic theory.

Increasingly with myself and with clients I pared away narrative, excluding emotion and movement from what we initially focused upon, namely, ultimately, the examination of held-energy systems. Now, though I listen "peripherally" to client history, I do not particularly want to begin by hearing my client's "story;" and I am surprised how many clients are relieved by that. "Thank God you are not going to get caught thinking the telling of my story is gong to make any difference," they say.

While I do ask about abuse incidents, as a focusing strategy I no longer request initially extended detail about actual situations which may be what the trauma is about, or when the pattern was laid in. Those details encompass incidental insights, strategies, not case history facts, which emerge soon enough, but not with traditional weight for me or for the client.

Unlike regular therapeutics, I offer an alternate strategy based upon the intuition that dissolution of the pattern occurs by focusing at levels which the verbal telling at best imitates. Cognitive and emotional integration may occur after the held-energy system is approached energetically; and this can be completed in more traditional talk therapies.

We do not have to quarrel or mediate about responsibility—which is an issue to be set aside, not fixedly, verbally determined. Brain appears actively engaged in solving the problem of traumatic immobility, and the balance of responsibility is delineated somewhat automatically as preverbal comprehension is manifest. What I try to *educate* my clients about is how the life energy can be held by trauma process and how its remobilization can be facilitated and witnessed. This requires a flexibility, not with words and insights, but rather with the vibrational levels themselves.

I believe there is a place for what fundamentalism is, but not where most mind/brains currently scan, in narrative forms, idea/belief systems, and their apposite accommodations, symbols. In this sense, fundamentalist phenomena reflect held-energy systematics, not narrative levels of incarnation.

Witnessing the energy as neurochemistry and vibration may offer not only the opportunity for fundamentalism to be properly, preverbally located, but it avoids the pitfalls of its misuse at ideational levels. It provides a direction for what to do with held energy, namely to dissolve its systems and to restore brain to its full energetic, healing capacities. That is perhaps why fundamentalists trust absolute qualities, because they intuitively identify thereby where brain is stuck.

Life Energy

Building upon the Reichian lineage, my own experiences, and those with clients, I saw our life energy as subtle, erotic, outward-moving, compassionate, empathic, loving, self-regulating, eager to respond and to adapt, sacred, creative, and playful. Under slowly overpowering or radically sudden stimulus, the mindbody neurochemically hardens, like the opossum feigning death, playing 'possum, while grabbed in the jaws of a coyote.

The opossum remains in the coyote's jaws in a deep, super trance-like state, without even the hint of energetic movement, much less physical movement. If the life force manifests, the jaws of the coyote will close involuntarily upon the presence of energy in the body of the opossum, killing it; *nothing personal.*

When the coyote drops this immobilized and uninteresting lump of flesh, and moves away, the opossum comes out of its neurochemical holding system and safely departs the scene. The immobilization which the opossum enters is then completed in a restoration of an active fight-or-flight set of responses, and the living opossum continues.

Levine and others claim that humans get stuck in this immobilization phase, resulting in anxiety and stress, as well as a lot worse, including permanent impairment of the ability to move and defend oneself. By extrapolation, entire hormonal neurochemistries can be held, and developmental sequences locked in inconclusion, waiting like Prometheus for Hercules to release them.

As passenger in the front seat of an automobile, we forget to fasten our safety belt, and our car hits a wall. Heading in *pre-windshield* chaos toward the windshield, our mindbody rigidifies in some energetically essential place in primitive brain, objectifying itself, becoming molecularly rigid, like, perhaps, the object it is about to hit.

Our life energies, including the auric, appear to immobilize *prior to* and *within* the moment of contact with the windshield. Let us suppose that we smash through the windshield with relative safety, get our cuts and bruises taken care of, and go on with our life in a coping, rehabilitative way. In one portion of the encoded memory of the pre-hitting-the-windshield situation, some supervisory energetic function of our mindbody presumably scans this section of held energy roughly ten times a second, even though we had the accident months or years ago.

This memory has not the flexibility of ordinary recall. Rather than "frozen," I prefer to think of this encoded memory as *held*, because the way out of the conundrum seems to be to hold again. Still, I find myself using "locked" at times, though this usage invites the image of penetrating the system with a key which the unlocker has, which is not what I think happens when the deepest kind of change occurs.

The energy within our primitive brain seems not to know what to do with this neurochemical traffic bump and detours around it. The rest of the neurochemistry is OK, yet as in Jesus' parable, the shepherd brain does not worry about the many sheep safe in the fold. It hunts for the one sheep that is lost.

Craziness, Toxicity, and Energy

Without this protective holding, the original flowing, perhaps chaotic pre-windshield energetic situation in the passenger's mindbody would allow the individual to float in cellular, metabolic openness. Without resistance to its momentum through the windshield, probably the integrity of the mindbody would be even more compromised, even destroyed. This experience of traumatic neurochemical immobility and the information it holds, hastily and radically processed, appears sealed when our neurochemical holding mechanism is so suddenly evoked by the accident.

The gates to this stored memory phenomenon, now a held-energy system, with all of its kinesthetic network of total body and mind involvement, are as if closed. The brain cannot enter its own locked, excuse me, closet, and as with a taboo, the remaining life energies appear to be forbidden to enter the room of encapsulated memory. Behind its door is some sense of chaos or pain which the mindbody cannot deal with. Our inner emotional sense is that without this neurochemical gateway to past overwhelm sealed, our circuits will burn out or we will go crazy, go over the edge, or "lose it."

I have come to think it is this *pre-windshield* sense of neurochemical disorder which is the only *craziness* there is. All the other usages of that word are a kind of elaboration. Everything else labeled "crazy"—eccentricity, odd behavior, word salad, etc.—could be a protection against sensing, or better, traversing that disorder, which is natural, both the disorder and the attempt to protect against it.

In this sense, for ourselves, we can never *be* crazy; we can merely *feel* crazy when we are in that pre-windshield phenomenon. What we term crazy in others or ourselves, including the phenomena of so-called psychosis, may be seen as tracer, dissociative, narrative spin-offs proposed by our brains in denial of the impossibility of processing this held, forbidden toxicity.

Like a circuit-breaker, the neurochemical process in our trauma mechanism both disrupts and protects, initially. When the remaining flowing energy cannot "find" or flow through the mindbody sequence of the trauma-instilled held-energy system, it also chemically denies access to the entry door, behind which there is indirectly perceived some sign of commotion, some variation on intense sensation. I think it is the mindbody's erotic "drive" to find its way into this forbidden kingdom juxtaposed with its inability to do so which causes our suffering and attendant, altered behavior and neurophysiognomy which we often sense as craziness, disease, or dysfunction in ourselves and in others.

To watch the energy might seem to require our witnessing it in some fixed pattern only, even hardened into stone-like "forms." Yet that is not the same as watching it in creative homeostasis, with clarity. Does the energy need to be fixed to see it? I don't think so. Clients and I have discovered we can manifest a manner of holding awareness which has a creative dwelling-upon focused quality which hovers apart from the energy and allows it to be. Our internalized parenting patterns try to shape the energy and determine it, yet to do so is to lose something critical for our healing process.

It is interesting how myths and psychologies end up focusing upon this central mindbody phenomenon, and we describe it in similar ways. One characterization of our traumatic closure might be a parable in the mode of Kafka, the master portraitist of trauma and dissociation.

The first time the mindbody scans, the chemical door to trauma-held memory is shut; the second time it is sealed. The third time, our erotic, scanning energy asks, "Where is the door? It was here just a moment ago." And the neurochemical doorkeeper replies, "What door? What are you talking about?" Meanwhile within/behind some such boundary, inside the held-energy system, there is conflict or chaos. Here is a neurochemical immobility within which is held the pre-windshield turbulence which the mindbody cannot master except by a diversionary end-run classically called *denial*.

And the mindbody and the energy which is the brain as well as what passes through it, appears to "want" nothing more than to get the energy moving again in precisely this stuck place. Whether there is actually a flow or that is the way it seems from within is unimportant. Brain knows something is wrong because it senses some portion as stuck. The information that the trauma contains cannot be quickly sorted, as it has been laid in too suddenly under disorienting compression of time and even body structure.

Though the event occurred years ago, we are still being hurtled through the windshield. And the signals of stuckness to the so-called conscious personality are announced in the form of unassailable patterns, addictions, suffering, and pain, all of which are complex and apparently, and frustratingly, immoveable.

This skewed compression may be observable at various levels, in structure, tissue, membrane, cell, and molecule, at subtle energetic levels (aurae) as well as, of course, the ideational and psychological states which convey them to our so-called consciousness. These held-energy system sites appear ultimately resolvable at a neurochemical level of organization whose subsequent inner homeostasis may be perceived as energetic by us, its "inhabitants." We again feel whole.

Superstition

We read the distress and our energetic approach and avoidance of the held energy within our subtle energy organization in narrative terms, with symbol, memory, cognition and the like. And we are unprepared when these modalities, these reflections, these imitations (*mimēsis*), if you will, of the energy do not yield real movement. After all, we sense, if we cannot trust our own experience as it presents to us, whose can we trust? Yet our own experience may come in forms that are secondary, not primary, nor close to the point of origin we are hunting for. We hover in the absoluteness of language and ideas long after they have lost their usefulness, even within a sentence, or a word.

Meanwhile, as in the classic experiment where a pigeon ritually bows and scrapes to influence randomly offered pellets of food, we are oscillating toward and away from the held-energy systems, trying to manipulate the secondary forms called insights and ideas, but never resolving the impasse from which, "defensively," they are generated as a response. With exquisite accuracy, Plato's allegory of the cave describes this traumatic, tragic situation, illustrating the difficulty of moving out of dissociation into enlightenment.

No wonder we are superstitious, for that is what *superstition* is, an attempt to solve a problem established at a primary energetic level by the secondary means of juxtaposing symbol, language, memory, and cognition. We use highway signs to tell us where we are, but the road determines where we go. No wonder the manipulation of these secondary imitations, superstitions, never reliably leads to real change, the dissolution of held-energy systems within our neurochemistries. That superstitions are recurrent and repetitious should tell us something.

This dissolution, I believe, is the area described by Aristotle's serious action, which consists of focusing upon an *inaction* leading to revised, trauma-free, *right action*, the only action in town. We could argue that Aristotle is concerned with how tragedy is an artistic form whose main focus is dissociation, an imitation of the energetic, not real, right action.

In the traumatic mechanism, strata of cellular, molecular, and subtle energy patterns appear laid in, incarnated if you will, in our mindbody-energy sequence.   Once they are held, they become cellularly, muscularly, and characterologically dominant pathways, river and riverbed, in the flowing of our life energy.

Where there is active flow, we can experience a sense of cellular and molecular openness, which can be perceived by itself, but also can be translated into unrestricted movement—physical, intellectual, characterological, emotional, and spiritual.   Thakar proposes significantly that we then can feel whole and, without ego, we can respond relationally to the world.

At base, our mindbody seems to want nothing more than to have lifted off the burden of its own rigidities, externally imposed as well as self-perpetuated. Primitive brain, especially in traumatic process, appears confounded by the speed, the invisibility with which these held-energy systems are set in. Because they are laid in at a complex interface between so-called self and the unyielding, so-called abusive environment, we become particularly alert about responsibility and how that is ascribed and delineated.

When the trauma pattern has been dissolved into, for lack of a better term, understanding (*cf.* Coleridge on Reason and Understanding), the energy flows and our heretofore compelling concern with boundaries is not a concern, nor is vigilance required. In fact, this energetic reworking (or, in Levine's original term, "renegotiation") is our brain's only task: to restore balance, vibrancy, and passionate equilibrium.   Clients and I have seen this self-monitoring, self-disciplining, homeostatic experience occur in a matrix where all possible permutations of energy are self-boundarying without seeming to impose or limit.

The life energy, which can be witnessed, is self-witnessing, is delicate and also powerful, beyond ordinary imagination. Traditional views of the nature of power may be radically challenged by our direct inner experience of transformation within the energetic reworking of held-energy systems. The implications for what to focus upon in difficult situations within a person's experience or in the outer world are significant, to say the least.

Our mindbody can view its own energetic process at a number of levels. At its least effective, least helpful level, it can remark upon the energy invested in the body with such comments as "I have a headache," and "It hurts here." Not only that, but the mindbody can accurately describe and enter the traumatic mechanism and heal itself (self so-called) by focusing upon the held-energy systems in a kind of steady, slightly shifting purview, and then by watching what happens.

Black and the Subtle Energies

Ultimately, upon this kind of viewing, a grid or point of energetic immobilization appears at the root or origin of each emerging, hoping-to-be-resolved pattern which some aspect of brain recognizes within its experience as shape and color. Clients and I have observed how this information somehow signals to the mindbody the nexus of a held-energy system.

Unlike the strategies of practitioners who deal with color variations within the spectrum, for held-energy systems, I think the significant "color" is **black**, where there is no vibration, no subtle energetic movement. The energy is *held*. I have found it interesting how few of the commentaries on chakra or other color healing systems pay attention to this, to me essential "color" phenomenon. Reich, an exception, identified its importance and, Sharaf reports, apparently could recognize its non-energetic presence in people, commenting to individuals, "You look black."

Theorists suggest that the original self-protective energies surrounding what has been called the fight-or-flight mechanism get frozen in trauma, and that these vectors need to be allowed to renegotiate their way into wholeness again, so that individuals may proceed with their lives with full, flexible armamentaria.

Among others, Levine posits that there are levels of entry into the trauma mechanism. As facilitators, we must move slowly into the memory system which contains the disruptive, toxic material, titrating, diluting at symbolic, meaning, motoric, and other levels. He calls the traumatic core center "T-*zero* [T_0]," the neurochemical center of the trauma memorial, as it were. Here, presumably, all things which need processing finally can be neurochemically slowed down and "witnessed," or processed and integrated by brain.

Traditionally, this point of origin may be located in two conflicting time frames:

a. the original moment when the trauma mechanism sets in, the pre-windshield moment, and

b. the point of access in current time when recollection entry to that original moment system is decodable.

Because in dissociation both moments are mixed, and the vectors of time often impossibly scrambled, approaching the point of origin as vibration through color and shape circumvents this historical conundrum. We can focus on what is puzzling brain presumably at the neurochemical level of information, not the narrative. How is this done?

My understanding is that our scanning mindbody identifies the point of origin in the traumatic patterning vibrationally as *black*, and I shall discuss black in detail in Chapter Two. At this point, suffice it to say that black appears the most important experience for what might be called our primitive brain, as black apparently signals a direction to avoid, and in the healing process, a direction for brain to attend to.

Unlike void black, which also occurs, black here is the black more of physics, than of art. It is not really even a color, but a state outside of vibration, hence out of time, containing within an held-energy system all potential of color and movement. Perhaps because it resembles the immobilities of death, the life force appears to "flow" around it or is pushed away from its penumbra.

This black can show different qualities (hard, soft, liquid, mottled, gray variations—again, see Chapter Two), depending upon the degree to which our mindbody "understands" its own held-energy systems. For example, at the edge of the core, the black often takes on characteristics of hardness, rectilinear planes, with a matte, dull surface. It seems these configurations place our mindbody close to the center of the held-energy system.

Getting to the historical point of origin of the trauma as memorialized may be locating the cause of our trauma, but it seems getting to the black locates the cause of our suffering as well as the point of origin of our narrative. When paying attention at the narrative level does not change the pattern, we can focus at a vibrational level upon the black.

The Healing Traditions

In the history of man's thought and attempt to heal, we have seen how our mindbody can enter the psychodynamic, kinesthetic, verbal, cognitive, and even imagery realms to resolve the impasses created by the traumatic mechanism. At base, however, the patterns will not resolve until our mindbody reaches the tolerance level of pure energy, beyond Plato's Forms. Here emotion, rationality, imagination, and cognition are seen as manifestations of traumatic patterning, or ego, rather than the "problem's" source.

This source appears stored ultimately at the subtle energy level surrounding and permutating the mindbody, and hence is invisible to ordinary awareness. In current shorthand, where trauma has not been resolved at the denser incarnate levels of meaning and plot, we witness the invisible so-called aura to see how and where the denser patterns are stored and generated. And by this strategy, witnessing is what we have to do. Brain does the rest.

Many of the clients I see have tried many forms of therapy, and the residual patterns they are working with have not been removed. These people are often experienced and comfortable with many strategies in various combinations: nutrition, acupuncture, faith healing, psychotherapy, psychodrama, psychoanalysis, diamond therapy, Reiki, yoga, meditation, etc. Yet in effect they all complain, "I have tried everything, but I can't get this pattern out."

Traditional practitioners may lead clients into a place of disgruntled and often exhausted acceptance that there is nothing they can do about their situation, which itself is a partial, and neurochemical, adjustment of sorts. At its darkest, this accommodation depends upon our generating secondary neurotransmitter opiates to sequester pain, like the daily numbing out of a toothache, and is best described by Thoreau as life of "quiet desperation," or by Freud as "normal neurosis."

The One-Third Rule

If we use a mindbody strategy, at some point we can view experience as spirit (Spirit) progressively densifying into our mortal, final flesh. When we want to witness the Godhead, we get as close to an unobstructed view of that mystery as we can. We go to that which is prior to the smallest perceivable, recordable phenomenon, and ask, "What is it that is the causal point of origin of that, say charming quark?" and we respond, "Spirit, or God." In this sense incarnation might show the following "descent": God/Spirit, sub-atomic elements/energy, atoms, neurochemistry/electromagnetic field, neurochemistry/molecules, cells, tissue, organs, structure. Parallel to these physical densities can be included fundamentalist convictions, emotions, ideas, body images, personality traits, and personality.

Our collective statistical wisdom notes that no matter what we do therapeutically, one third of us stays the same, one third gets better, one third gets worse. We know that these partial curing rates can be achieved by focusing at the denser levels of energy "incarnation," where the particular pattern seems to originate and be lodged. These include our organs, tissues, bones, and the overt neurochemistries, including their manifestations as emotions.

This is not a bad batting average, for it implies two-thirds of us not getting worse. Yet for the intractable patterns, and for a comprehension of the point of origin which conceivably could lead not to a one-third, or two-thirds, rule of accommodation but to a much higher success rate of actual healing, we may be able to get comfortable gradually with levels of energetic density acknowledged in the presence of so-called *subtle energies*. These are what appear to hold and determine the interaction between mind and body and channel movement of spirit into greater densities of incarnation. They are considered to reside throughout all the levels of incarnation and to connect them.

That our mindbody can gain quick and potent access to these levels by focusing on the vibrational patterns through color has not been easily understood, except perhaps in the world of art. Nor easily understood are the strategies or blocks, resistances, which keep us from entering the color realm, once we are in traumatic process. In the past, such attempts have required taking leave of traditional verbal and ideational modes of structuring experience, and entering spacey realms of arcane, "woo-woo" ritual and hocus-pocus, and, in short, going off the deep end.

In my own case, it has taken decades to acclimate to this energetic level while remaining functioning in the "ordinary" world. And I keep forgetting that fact when I enthusiastically invite clients into these experiences, as if it should be as easy for them as it is for me, now that after decades I myself have finally cusped into a new, and old, awareness.

Our brain memorizes and negotiates the complex information contained in the trauma "surround" in vibrational energetic frequencies, in color, odor, (musical) sound, taste, touch and intuition. Thus, at some primitive brain level, specific imagery, as one might have in daily life, or in a dream, fantasy, or recollection of the past, seems ultimately irrelevant to the resolution of the held-energy system.

We can spend thirty years in Jungian therapy analyzing dreams and never move the basic pattern. Sometimes there is an exception when, in laborious ways, and by serendipitous chance, we stumble across a cure or healing resolution. For Freud, his vision of his own trauma resolution, delineated in *Civilization and Its Discontents*,

Moses and Monotheism, etc., seems to be that for all his psychoanalytic work on himself, he was not at the bottom of the personal, ethnic, and cultural patterns which bothered him. He appears to come to only an accommodation of sorts with his suffering.

My guess is that, like many of us, he entered his traumata, his tragic patterns, at the analytic level. This was a defensive "rescue station" from the implications of patterning in himself which were traumatically sealed at the energetic levels, some of which he perceived (*cf.* his commentaries on libido and sexuality) and attempted to manipulate "rationally," through verbal centers of the brain by so-called analysis.

Freud's split with Reich over working with the vibrational body and the energetic Freud once saw, places Freud well within a classical human lineage (*cf.* commentary on Moses, Chapter Seven), where the spiritual hero accesses the energetic and channels it into stone, a recurrent human dilemma. Not an easy man, and without supports and with antagonism and fear directed at himself, Reich may have appropriated the toxicity of his own patterning and, evaluated increasingly mad, died. Sharaf reports that Reich's end was not marked by a lack of lucidity or connection, so the sadness and isolation of his story is profound.

Energy System Reconfigures

As Freud and other analysts intuited, and haphazardly saw in their clients at best on a one-third success basis, the held-energy system, or pattern, can be viewed by our mindbody. Under the insight I have garnered, the black energy hiatus is allowed to be held, to dissolve, remobilize, and the vibrational information within, *i.e.*, the colors, to reconfigure.

What if developmental sequences have been suspended in one portion of the brain or in some cellular sequences throughout our mindbody by the circumscribing of radical traumatizing experience into, as it were, its Noah's ark of a held-energy system? Within trauma reconfiguration, these sequences could be then molecularly, neurochemically integrated until a vibrant and mobile, erotic, homeostatic calm permeates all levels of experience. At the emotional level, where there was despair, there can now be hope.

The held-energy systems represent our mindbody's attempt to limit the damage of the pre-windshield over-stimulation and challenge. Characteristically, apparently within that trauma mechanism, our brain produces a "big bang" phenomenon, wherein the original wholeness of our energetic mindbody is quickly divided (shattered may be our inner experience of this abrupt division) into a universe of discreet, seemingly "whole" planetary fragments. The mechanism thus resembles burying the household silver in small parcels throughout the plantation to protect the family heritage and wealth, in the face of Sherman's advancing, life-annihilating troops.

In the sweep of the post big-bang phenomenon, our mindbody appears to bolt the planetary pieces together, in muscularly rigid, characteristic, characterological patterns of holding, personality types, etc. These narratives often seem to demonstrate themselves energetically in a literal black grid pattern, like a magnified section of a screen door, or, in a more flexible rendering, a net (*cf.* Aeschylus' *Agamemnon*).

A Solution

As I tried to expand my understanding of the additive nature of these *narratives*, I returned to classic texts I had studied and taught then for decades to understand how held-energy systems conclude. At the level of ordinary awareness, like the gestalt of Odysseus/Telemachus/Penelope after the Trojan War, in trauma we are left picking up the pieces of our experience, or casting out and drawing in a "net," gathering the parts, whose sequence is called a *pattern* or even a *narrative*, before a neurochemical resynthesis can occur, and the energy can flow again.

Interestingly, plot, as we know it in plays, myths, and stories, deconstructs thus into the energetic by abandoning the language centers of the brain. Brünnhilde rides her horse onto Siegfried's flaming funeral pyre, and the gods and their place, Valhalla, conclude; it is a fiery and thus I think perhaps somewhat suspect completion. Describing trauma resolution as violent, or with violent imagery, risks retraumatization and, I believe, keeps us from crucially witnessing the erotic nature of the life force.

As noted before, I find it intriguing how our understanding of tragic depths is weaned on tragedies whose plots conclude approaching the (black) bottom, bringing us to a Good Friday total eclipse, where we need to be before we can witness spontaneous movement. And we leave the theater at that point. Over time, I have become more interested in the for me more difficult bottoming out and up, as it were. I want to see the moment turning from total eclipse to the first reappearance of the sun's corona.

Again, Aristotle terms most tragic (*tragictatus*) the non-extant tragedy about Merope, the mother who is about to kill a young stranger, recognizes him as her son and does not kill him. Likewise, Abraham does not kill Isaac, and in a variation on the same theme, the dead Jesus is resurrected. Energetically, I think the latter situation describes a chemistry of traumatic resolution witnessed from within, while the former reveals how such transformation looks when acted in the real world.

Commandingly, Aeschylus' *Oresteia* reveals the same tragic movement (*metabasis*) out of traumatic immobility, when the Furies are transformed into the Eumenides, the Peaceful Ones. We may witness Good Saturday's moment, our Harrowing of Hell, our descent into bardo, and, at the point of origin (*To*), crucially, our *turning*, just prior to Resurrection.

Movement and Change

Ultimately this energetic resynthesis can occur at a matter-of-fact level, and the narrative of the original trauma can be matter-of-fact, detailed, and not filled with racing or stolid affect. Freud and other healers, and most individuals, have recognized this creative narrative in therapeutic process, in art, drama, and the like.

Homer's *Odyssey* is an example of such a journey, taking place within a single circuit of our self-scanning mindbody. Each event sequence in Odysseus' journey home, his encounters with the Cyclops, the Sirens, etc., characterizes a traumatic fragment, as compelling and absorbing as an entire planet. Yet because they are set within a dissociative framework, the dislocations of the Trojan War, these sequences are ultimately incomplete, and Odysseus continues his journey homeward.

There is a more fundamental reality expressed at Ithaca, Odysseus' home, which occurs simultaneously with and split off from his adventures with, for example, the Sirens. This pattern is ultimately confronted in the "slaughter" of the fragments, Penelope's suitors, who seek to replace the lost Odysseus. Within this strategy, the Odysseus is itself a traumatic fragment or "planet," with all its attenuated grandiosity and collapse, linked as fragment to other fragments by Odysseus' characterization as wily or clever.

In the slaughter of the suitors we see the formation of a gestalt, an *e pluribus unum*, if you will, where the plural fragmentation of suitors is reduced to the unitary figure of Odysseus. I think such gestalt formulation is similar to the development of a single protagonist out of the plurality of the Greek tragic chorus, or the figure of New Testament Jesus as personality gestalt of the Old.

After reconnecting with Penelope and Telemachus, the Odysseus continues with the pattern in a transformation of subtle energy. He paradoxically heads inland carrying his oar upon his shoulder, vowing to set it down when he meets someone who does not know what he is carrying.

At some important level, at the conclusion of the *Odyssey*, a significant subtle energy pattern has been revised, and we may see something of what serious movement looks like. While the Aristotelian concern with change (*metabasis*) does not specify what kinds of change, I think we could make a case for differentiating activity, movement, and change at the energetic level on the lines that the early episodes of the *Odyssey* are the equivalent of ordinary therapeutic release. Such release is a temporary relief from our held pattern and a precursor of movement, but does not take the pattern out entirely. The sequences of plot on the order of what happens next are mere activity.

Change would then mean the complete dissolution of the held-energy pattern into the vibrant information of *clear*, which does not occur at the end of the *Odyssey*, though the promise of healing is there. At its conclusion, we are given a glimpse of the proper attitude toward facing the black—paradoxical, respectful, undaunted by absurdity or narrative logic.

Oedipus at Colonus

I think our dissolution of our holding patterns is more completely described at the end of Sophocles' *Oedipus at Colonus*, where Oedipus is preparing to die. Everyone who formerly rejected him suddenly wants to possess what he is, his power and knowledge, having endured and experienced the taboos he has enacted. Only Theseus, ruler of Athens, asks the Oedipus (the pattern) how and under what conditions he(it) wants to die. It is Theseus who protects him from the assaultive objectifying functions of the brain, his warring sons, his brutalizing former brother-in law King Creon, which try to get rid of the held-energy system he embodies.

It is Theseus who critically does not tell Oedipus what he must or must not do. Rather he asks the Oedipus, the held-energy system, in effect, "What needs to happen here?" Then Oedipus responds, saying he wants to die, at Colonus, with Theseus to protect him. Oedipus goes into the grove at Colonus with Theseus, and his transformation occurs invisibly.

This absence of density seems to me appropriate to approaching the black held-energy system as source of suffering as well as point of origin of activity for most of us. When the energetic information is absorbed, Oedipus is energetically transformed and disappears, leaving only the Theseus part of the gestalt. At this point, activity ceases, and action begins.

This every one of us heard him say,
And then we came away with the sobbing girls.
But after a little while we withdrew
We turned around—and nowhere saw that man,
But only the king, his hands before his face,
Shading his eyes as if from something fearful,
Awesome and unendurable to see.
Then very quickly we saw him do reverence
To Earth and to the powers of the air,
With one address to both.
                              But in what manner
Oedipus perished, no one of mortal men
Could tell but Theseus. It was not lightning,
Bearing its fires from Zeus, that took him off;
No hurricane was blowing.
But some attendant from the train of heaven
Came for him; or else the underworld
Opened in love the unlit door of earth.
For he was taken without lamentation,
Illness or suffering; indeed his end
Was wonderful if mortal's ever was.

                              trans. Robert Fitzgerald

Blake and Historical Memory

It appears that our so-called ego and its attendant personality fragments do not give up until they leave entirely the narrative levels of experience organization. In the writings of Hegel and those who draw on him, even the promise of sustained ecstasy can be historically dissolved into energetic flow. History, a function of trauma and retraumatization as we currently assemble it, ceases to be, as memory is freed and transmuted into pure(r), clear, and right movement. At least that is our intuition.

From this perspective, the history of the study of trauma is the study of historical memory, which itself is the study of forms which the trauma mechanism produces. These include all art, politics, and thought. Not that speech, and its spin-off, language, need to be considered as a derivative of trauma, incapable of occurring without trauma's platform. Yet four factors suggest their narrative, peripheral nature.

First, thought appears adjunctive to the removal of held-energy systems. In our sessions, we place ourselves in the inner energetic landscapes and witness. Second, in terms of the fight-or-flight mechanism, for the most part, speech seems irrelevant. Third, in terms of relational eros, language may modulate, but it does not necessarily determine intercourse. Fourth, language often exists in linear time, perpetrating and perpetuating linear time as a function of grammar and syntax.

The energy immobilized in trauma, in its contained forms, appears to filter and intermingle into the sounds which emerge as speech, so that it is difficult to see where trauma and speech at many different levels are not coincident. Blake examines this coincident differentiation in his *Songs of Innocence and Experience*, where the relationship between Innocence and Experience may be seen to oscillate upon paradoxical fulcra between untraumatized energy and that which is contained in the offspring of the trauma mechanism, the held-energy system.

Where we view our conduct without awareness of the trauma which perpetrates its activity form, we can be considered innocent. Where we reenter the held-energy system, we are also innocent, but by doing that we pass into experience, including chaotic experience and the possibility of chaotic experience as well as of its resolution. We acknowledge our self-healing powers. Where we realize we must stop retraumatizing ourselves and stop perpetrating trauma upon others, our innocence is based upon the fact that our "experience" is not fluid, but held.

Experience, in this sense, is ultimately conducted upon a trauma-free landscape which involves innocence as the vigilant modality with which we dissolve the Moby Dick of our trauma. But to accomplish this clarification, we become experienced. Our experience, transforming us, is of reestablishing energetic flow, innocence, by our engagement with held energy.

The recognition that we are caught in held-energy patterns which resist completion certainly takes us beyond ignorance to places of experience wherein we can restore the innocent, clear energetic. Likewise, our understanding of innocence and experience is confounded by recognition that our activities are promulgated by traumatic patterning. Those who sing know that there is an interface where energy and the denser vibrations of words and music meet which can generate a transcendent experience, exposing vistas beyond form, beyond holding, and beyond and within innocence.

CHAPTER THREE: ON BLACK

Integrity

When we have dissolved the patterns, what does the new, old integrity look like? Cycles of continuation, addiction, shame, guilt, and forgiveness all may be seen as emotional approximations of the energy unsuccessfully attempting to approach and dissolve the black held-energy sites of immobilization. In contradistinction, integrity has a cellular openness and even liveliness which suggests completion within each moment, a blending of Blake's vision of Innocence and Experience. Thakar describes such integrity as ego-less, undivided wholeness.

In these portions of our brain/chemistry, where before there seemed to be compression, determinism, fate, and destiny, we may now experience the neurochemistry of clear hope, possibility, and, interestingly enough, responsibility. These hallmarks of maturity have been recognized, perhaps with wistful longing, by psychodynamic therapists.

Boundary confusions and rigidities which we experience consciously as part of ourselves and those around us are evoked from within held-energy systems and appear signs of traumatic positioning. When we are centered, the energy flows, inward and outward and compassionately, ready like the Christ, to take on the Other patterns of pain for the world, in order to solve or resolve them. Here the (Christ) child says to the world, including significantly its parents, "Let me absorb the stuck places you perpetrate onto me, and I'll solve them with my energetic capacity. I return them to you healed and completed, so you and we can be free."

The psychiatrist Bion describes a function which each mother provides for its child, namely the capacity to act as a predigestor for the child's raw experience. Like the Eskimo mother who chews the blubber for its child and deposits it in the infant's mouth, so mothering has a quality of somehow taking on the difficult energetics of the child's experience and redepositing them into the child's being in digestible order. "You want your diaper changed," says Eskimo mom to her fidgety infant.

But what if the infant provides a similar *sacerdotal* capacity for the parent? What if within the symbiotic interrelationship at an energetic level the infant absorbs important information, including parental traumata which are visited upon or intuitively pressed upon or within, say, the auric field of the child? Child/parent reciprocity is truncated by the nature of trauma transmission, active and permeative; for as infants our education into the world is as both student and teacher.

The Speed of the Trauma Mechanism

Not only in its initial evocations to protect the mindbody in crisis, but once in place, the rapidity of the appearance of the held-energy system defies what we think of as awareness. There is no lag time, no lead time. Precipitously, invisibly set in our neurochemistry, its manifestation in the so-called psychopathology of daily life is instantaneous. Its invocation occurs before whatever our self-awareness is can notice it. And because it propels us outside of vibration, it exists outside of human, historical time.

The war is started and completed in the same moment, and we are remaindered to exist, sorting rubble and narrative artifacts—disease, addictions, theological disputations—thinking we are doing something when in fact our personal, ethnic, cultural patterns never change, nor, so perceived, can they. At least not the ones which we continue to perpetrate. The cycles of war and peace remain unpredictable and predictable, as we are condemned to repeat the historical, ethnic, religious, and personality patterns we have taken on before we knew their impossibilities. Is not our lesson to learn how they are laid in, how to dissolve them, and how to sustain the resultant freedom? Might this be progress?

Trust and Trauma

In conditions of trauma, our brain, or the section of our brain which is involved, apparently recognizes only two things, trust and trauma. The millisecond trust is offered, or achieved, even in the most grotesquely similar forms to the original traumatic configurations, the held-energy system is offered up for healing. I intuit it is our mindbody's recognition of similarity of traumata patterning in the other person which "causes" marriage and ultimately divorce, bonding and separation. For when the initial honeymoon platform of trust is established, the marriage and our healing must begin.

I think we marry to be healed, and divorce because we mistake the trauma offered in response to trust by ourself and our spouse as the ultimate, dead-end truth. This "truth" of separation, offered by each partner in trauma, reveals everything—personality, aspiration, and behavior—as stuck and eternally immobilized, rather than an opportunity for mobility and healing. "I can no longer tolerate my husband's drinking," the wife explains to the divorce counselor.

We, husband and wife, primitively assume that what is immobile in us and our consorts is bottom-line truth, when, as Buddhists might suggest, we are then most in illusion. Right action in response to the truth reflects reality, which is not, in an earlier sense, the truth.

Clients sometimes comprehend this mechanism when we view these two stages of the brain space-rocket, trust and trauma, or when they can see the interface of instantaneity as two abutting energetic and emotional "tectonic plates," with the crucial fault line running between them, and sometimes down the middle of their brain, fundamentally in the somewhere between left and right.

Our mindbody misreads this rending interface as failure. When trust is offered, the next phase to be brought forth, instantaneously as well as over a long time, is the trauma, in the form of dissociative behavior and its denser expression in dissociative patterning within the so-called personality of the partner.

Dissociation

Dissociative behavior has two features. First, it demonstrates our mindbody's traumatic pattern, in often disguised form. Second, it demonstrates our brain's problem of not having access to its own (crucial) material. The very neurochemical sealing brain institutes for its protection enforces a split or division which is painful, and confounding.

Our brain apparently experiences this self-sealing as an abandonment or dislocation of major proportions, and in the desire to reconstrue/reconstruct the energetic balance it somewhat vaguely recalls, it fractionates even further, stressing out our neurochemical situation. Our mindbody attempts to reevoke the original pre-windshield sequence, this time in order to *get it right* so we are not left with stuck debris as in the first moment of the initial trauma. By condoning this repetition—do we dare call it an imitation?—without completion, we merely coat *To* with overlay; this is *retraumatization*.

A client discovers the energy of nicotinic acid laid in prenatally by her smoking mother in a brown grey cloud. "This is where I start to want to light up," she reports.

" Enter a brown/black sub-particle of the cloud," I advise.

"Now it's as if I have lighted up."

"Cigarette companies aren't going to want to hear about this. Does brain know what needs to happen here?" I ask.

"No," she reports. After a while, she says, "This stuff is killing me; it's got to get out. In this place I know my mother loves me, but I don't know why she is killing me with this [stuff]." We discuss various ways to eliminate the toxicity, and she comes to the surface image with the cloud turned yellow, and considerable stress removed, a partial but considerable solution. She reports two days later that she has no further desire to smoke, a state she now has maintained for three years.

We see how fetal brain is confounded by the original trauma of the introduction of the acid into her system, and how her brain in dissociation is unable to do anything with this toxicity. Thus, superstitiously, brain repeats the intake of the acid by smoking, in order to create yet another opportunity. *This* time I'll get the original toxicity out. Because it cannot find the point of origin of the pattern located in the black, it addictively retraumatizes, passing by the hapless chemistry which stands by the road, muted in immobility.

It is this view of finding the potential for movement where there is none apparent which has given me hope about dissociative process, a phenomenon I have been intuitively concerned about since childhood. The term *dissociation* has entered the vocabularies of many educated people, and there are dangers in using the term too loosely. Yet the term describes a cluster of phenomena which move in usage from the very specific to a more general sense of disconnection in speech and behavior.

When clinicians talk about dissociation, they usually are referring to people who are vague, drifting off in their speech, spacey, and not connected to the immediate reality. People who are dissociated are characterized as split off from their feelings, fogged out, indistinct, not focused, not grounded, and not responsive. By a sort of contrast, in psychosis, these (perhaps) empty spaces are filled with delusions or hallucinations. Yet dissociation can refer to the client's inner experience of active stage memories coming forth in the contactive phase of therapy, or of numbing.

Dissociation can also be seen as the mechanism that engenders this splitting off, as our mindbody's way to respond to stress or the result of its response to stress. In this sense it may overlap or be identical with traumatic process, which rigidifies in a held-energy system. Dissociation is connected directly to the traumatic process of staying alive in the face of physical or psychological annihilation.

From an alternate point of view, in those moments of obvious fragmentation when people are spacey, what we may be seeing is toxicity, a variation of the greater dissociation manifest by everybody as just plain ordinary behavior, not something categorically worse. What is so interesting is that our dissociative process is not necessarily perceived by us as such from within.

Session Fallout

I had one client who engaged in a session with full agreement about what to anticipate, and made significant, even ebullient contact with some of his held-energy systematic. Three days later, when he experienced the toxicity surrounding the reworking at the energetic level, he claimed he felt retraumatized by the process. "I was in traumatic dissociation," he asserted, "You should have known that [and (presumably) altered your approach]."

What I found intriguing was that the client, prepared by me and his therapist for everything else about the work, was not prepared for the real change that the energy work evoked in him, even though we fully discussed his therapy network and how he was going to proceed after I departed his town. "I did not pay to experience confusion for the next week [a possibility we had discussed for its creative potential at some length]," he continued to express enragedly to his therapist.

His therapist, himself a victim of sexual abuse, found it difficult to process his client's response because of his own concerns with the rubric of retraumatization, and his declared desire to stand by his client. When I tried to negotiate this impasse, I was met with the client's refusal to meet with me to discuss the boundary issues. The therapist sensed he could not confront the issues at that point in the therapy, and expressed his frustration that our work had complicated, at least temporarily, his longer-term management of an obviously distressed client.

It seems our brain system can be surprised by its own power and structures. Some people, including me, need various decompression formats before we can test the mix as to what toxicity we can or cannot tolerate. In the above-mentioned encounter, in addition to the chagrin I felt because I had discussed at some length with the client these very issues, the additional irony was that this client presented himself as dissociated—syntactically, emotionally, a very unusual place to describe, even though dissociation and its sequellae are the reason people go into therapy to begin with.

The reportage from an experienced client who presents responsibly and claims after positive, prolonged engagement in the session that "I was dissociating" is claiming a responsibility for which there is syntactically slim possibility. Yet that is what everyone can say, and in various ways says all the time. The relationship of retraumatization to the initial uncovering of traumatic patterning must be strategized about with the client over time, and, as it were, collegially. Anticipating similar situations, I resolved to include the therapist as witness and support in any future sessions.

Increasingly, I found dissociation interesting to observe, particularly with those who are vigorously, cogently manifesting their trauma as reality, but whose movement between trust and trauma is instantaneous, shifting neurochemically between parts of a sentence, even a word. I proffered that everyone is in various stages of dissociation and dissociative toxicity. That became my initiating bottom line. Freud might have said, "You have rediscovered the unconscious."

For someone to say, "I am in dissociation," as if that were special, is equivalent to saying, "I am breathing" or "I am a sinner," both of which statements may express some truth. Perhaps the real issue is to identify the density or toxicity level of our dissociation. However, it is my experience that taking an interventionist approach toward controlling the toxicity by unilaterally determining how and when to intervene risks retraumatization. This is the place where the problem can be shared between practitioner and client: Could we ask, "What do you want me to do in light of your dissociative process?"

We casually talk a lot about "splitting," but neurochemically it is hard to achieve and hard to imagine, say, if you are God starting

from scratch with no intuition about how to divide. Yet the capacity
to differentiate one experience from another may be a part of the
mechanism which engenders our dissociative experience.

It seems important to offer this strategy to our mindbody as it
proceeds into the energetic and into our held-energy systems. Each
venture into a pattern may bring up on the screen(s) of so-called
consciousness emotion and other memories, but these are not
important to the healing process in a dwelling-upon sort of way. I
propose to the client these memories can be honored, or challenged,
played with "horizontally," in the form of relating details about the
situation recalled: "My father was wearing blue socks, and we went
to church every week that summer." But I intuit they are no
substitute for "vertical" entry into the held energetic of black.

The Brain Witnesses Itself

If we take the stance that until clear, everyone is in some
degree of dissociative process, how do we get the brain to see itself?
Descartes approaches the trauma mechanism in the same way that I
found myself doing with Jane Austen, by turning the meditation focus
upon itself. Yet the resultant Cartesian *cogito ergo sum* is a side order
of French-fried potatoes, not the *entrée*—a bit of linguistic pig iron off
the molten, from which all sorts of intriguing substructures can be, and
are, hung. As such, does it not merely reflect, imitate, or represent
some deeper, prior, energetic movement and its fallout? In Descartes'
Meditations, I see only one serious, energetic movement indirectly or
metaphorically acknowledged, and that is noted at the point of the
cogito. The remainder seems to be rationalization, elaboration, and
consolidation.

From our experience of myth and song, we know that the
language used to help us focus at the energetic level cannot be
ordinary language, at least not for the most part. The language used
must suggest its narrative and perpetrative function, as well as the
direct experience of the energetic, from which the client can pull away
as s/he finds words to describe what is invisible.

When working with clients at this level, I currently form my suggestions and commentary referring to *brain* and to *neurochemistry*. I think it is possible and creative to witness one's experience as brain and as neurochemistry, and that for a time, such witnessing may be necessary to help clients to scan their process, particularly as what they process is "presenting" in traumatic dissociation.

For this reason, I use the term *brain* to bring an alternative awareness to our dissociative awareness that we are a physical, neurochemical process. As carriers dwelling within dissociation, it is not surprising that we easily forget it.

Furthermore, if mind is some energetic form or surround of brain, to refer to its physiological nature brings mind into a new relationship with brain (not its source, but its density). That much of what mind thinks it is it is not, suggests the pervasive dissociative nature of our so-called consciousness.

Underneath mind's activity may lie a fundamentalist understanding of brain's physiology and its traumatic densities. That these are characterized as energetic hardnesses in black means we may, as it were, help mind to pass through its own fundamentalism, traumatically instilled. Its fluid life force is revealed much in the same way physicists reveal the electromagnetic particles which make up hard, black coal.

Black

I think it is *black*, seen, felt, sensed, or intuited, which provides entry into the base (*To*), the point of origin of held-energy systems. For black most often appears disturbing to our primitive brain at an energetic level. Clients repeatedly experience this phenomenon. All other colors express some vibrational movement. As in physics, black is held energy which does not move.

When we hang out energetically with the black, we discover the colors which reemerge, as our life energy saturates, reworks, and transforms the grid of held, immobilized energy. Could this understanding which leads us to conceive of additive black as containing all color, be correspondent with our experience of trauma?

The following are some intuitions drawn from my experience with clients who work with me at these levels.

Black. Energetic black itself can be described to have many qualities and textures: Smooth, vaporous, corrugated, wall-like, coal-like, jagged, jewel-like, ash-like, sooty, rough, dripping, or melting, depending upon the stages of resolution of the held-energy system. After a while, client and practitioner can get a feel for what brain is saying about the problem by the way the black system is graphically represented. If it is dense and hard, we may see brain "punning" on the neurochemical difficulty of the held-energy system, or rather its representation, because the visible form is always a step away from the invisible.

Training the brain to approach or seek out the black, rather than to move away from it, or to feel black scoot away when focus is placed upon it, is a marvelous and hope-inspiring faculty. It often appears as if we are stalking some prey, only the prey contains information which self-unlocks, once the proper etiquette for approach has been discovered.

The Particle Approach

If we go toward black, our brain may need to divide the system into smaller sub-particles until the pattern can be understood neurochemically and dissolved. This is a central strategy, and it is my experience that our brain can scan, and obviously does, to any level of magnification resolution in its system to discover where the trauma, or its equivalent, is. Why can't we join our journeying brain through greater ranges of density than heretofore we have thought possible?

If brain can resolve one particle, it can generalize and quickly resolve whole, linked archipelagoes of problematic areas. The impact of this strategy for cancers is already being probed at the neurochemical level by medical research, but not yet, to my knowledge, using this black strategy.

Our task becomes to discover to what level we must go to find a "particle" whose toxicity is tolerable and is decodable. I find that where the system stalls, or a fragment seems too stuck, I suggest that the client enter a sample area of the color of the fragment and again find a sub-particle, and tell me what its shape is.

Often the shape will not be the same as the "parent" fragment. Some are duplicating the parent form at each new level, which presents another problem, which I think has to do with not understanding this magnification strategy. One very experienced therapist complained, "But I have never done this sort of thing. I didn't know I could do this." I am not alone in proposing that our so-called awareness can go to many levels of magnification beyond what we normally think of as ourselves, to cellular, molecular, even sub-molecular levels.

I suppose (re)training our brain to approach the black is at the heart of those who attempt to master held-energy systems by dealing with "black magic." Controlling for the black in this "magic" way seems to me to miss the point, and to head us into all sorts of problems, especially having to do with power and control. At the center of all black configurations, hidden sometimes in places we would never look or think were important, we faithfully can find clear, sacred light.

From this perspective, evil, and its gestalt form of Satan, are the result of not comprehending the nature of traumatic black, and the difficulty brain has in approaching held-energy systems. Like the afore-mentioned famous superstitious pigeon in the experiment, the brain tries to figure out how it achieved relief from its own patterning, and ends up in dissociative behavior and thought patterns which are *superstition*. At times mind itself can be thought of as a trauma-related phenomenon.

From this point of view, professional lineages and so-called scientific approaches to the issues of disease and therapy might promote concealed superstitious behavior, wedded to narrative, something the scientific method is supposed to protect us from but cannot, because of the nature of the brain's avoidance of the demanding color black.

There are times when clients report they are in black and they feel safe there. This is another phase of the dissolving, for as long as the energy is held, our mindbody is protected from having to confront the pre-windshield chaos contained within the held-energy system. Whatever energetic black is—color, neurochemistry, or other process or capacity—with power to effect our configurations of stress and personality, it takes center stage.

Reich and Black Orgone

In the 1940s and 1950s, Wilhelm Reich identified the presence of deadly orgone, or black energy in the atmosphere, affecting weather and humans, the latter with disease. Utilizing similar insights to the ones considered here, Reich saw the deadly orgone as pervasive in our environment and influencing human experience.

Throughout his life, he focused upon trauma and its deadening effect on the body and its energies, and reportedly could see "black" energy in people. Myron Sharaf has told me that Reich would report his observation to people, including clients, saying, "You look black." Then he would ask them about how they felt, and talk with them about their feelings. He attempted many strategies to evoke dissolution of the armoring within the mindbody as well as in the environment, including those dealing with black, though to my knowledge, not the one offered here.

Black and Racism: A Digression

I wondered what connection if any there might be between the energetic black of trauma and our current naming our racially colored pinktans and browns as whites and blacks. It had seemed to me an act of great courage and genius for Malcolm X and others to begin showing how linguistically the odds had been stacked against Negroes because we pinktans called ourselves white, with all the advantageous rights and privileges entitled thereunto, while the Negroes were merely some alternative. The militant blacks of the 1960s argued, "If you are going to call yourselves white (good, pure, etc.), we shall name your game by calling ourselves black. And black is not bad; black is good."

It seemed to me the dangers of polarization incipient in the use of racist language and cloaked in intra- as well as interpersonal patterns of trauma and retraumatization in the form of social, personal, and physical abuses thus were rendered more syntactically visible. Blacks now faced their perpetrators and their own patterns in a way which at its best revealed deep schisms in the social fabric of the whites, for whites and blacks alike, though blacks were forced to see and experience these schisms from the down position, as they always had.

If we treat other people as objects, or as projections of our own sense of inferiority, what does that say about us? Why would anyone who is secure and balanced not treat another with respect, with equality, if only to manifest the Golden Rule? Within the continuing discussions and confrontations about race, our deepest holding patterns surfaced in obverse narrative form. We revaluated our freedom to vote, our right to have skin color and racial characteristics disregarded in public settings, and our right to equal opportunities.

A parallel set of retraumatizing holding patterns, *vis-á-vis* homosexuals, women, men, the homeless, the poor, various ethnicities, the mentally-ill, the disabled, those supporting the Psychological Reformation of the 1960s and 1970s, have all emerged, in politically correct and incorrect ways. Yet from my acquired perspective on trauma, I intuited that a fundamental issue in the traumatizations and retraumatizing structures of the social fabric of racism might occur at the level of trauma energetics. Simply, how does brain deal with the presence of black, as discovered within the held-energy systems of our mindbody?

Why does racism persist at subtle and unsubtle levels? So much has been accomplished, yet something sticks and resists clarification. By declaring themselves as "black," were African-Americans positioning themselves proximate with the invisible and unseen held-energy systems of the trauma mechanism itself? In terms of what they report experiencing, they might as well have been. Facing their black, we face ours.

With monolithic dog-headedness, I saw how the fundamental conundrum of held-energy spawns violence, superstition, rebellion, projective persecutions, and abuse. All of that does not belong with African-Americans any more than it does with any of the world-wide victim/perpetrator sequences which are still a tragic rule rather than a human exception. The lineages of abuse and victimization by whites in recent African-American history seem pervasive, yet the difficulty of finding a narrative solution through this morass has engendered rage, helplessness, and sadness in me.

To identify with the color black somehow, and not directly, may acknowledge that like everybody else, African-Americans have been traumatized by experience and dwell in trauma's immobilities. Like the Christ child, could the African-American confront a wounded white authority and take on the burden of its wounding? Baldwin, Angelou, and Malcolm X, among many others have described this process with moving force.

As someone presenting differently, any person may encounter projective scapegoating, providing externalized location for "white" trauma and retraumatizing capacities upon him or herself. I myself had known that growing up within so-called white society. Until we dissolve our patterns, we are instructed that adjustment to such abuse is what we call ordinary give and take of human socialization experience.

How much could claiming the color black for their own reflect blacks' aiming for the held-energy site of healing? I think every mindbody longs to achieve that site but cannot because of neurochemical, energetic prohibitions, skewing the approach and avoidance which has marked American responses to so-called issues of color. Paradoxically, this strategy may hold a real possibility of healing, if no further retraumatization occurs. I think only partial healing has occurred around this issue.

As chromatic variation on energetic movement, some pre-organic brown also may prejudice us toward retraumatizing as well as toward healing the "bruise." Tan or lighter brown energetically may suggest a greater lifting off of the black of trauma, yet it seems all color holds some attachment to personality. Black, here, by contrast, is qualitatively different, outside of vibration and time, and the shift from black to brown, from immobility to initial mobility, seems to me a qualitative, not merely quantitative transformation.

Even though lighter "black" may seem an improvement when working with held-energy systems, it is important to state the full trajectory so that there can be no misunderstanding or manipulation of the point of view I am developing here. *My goal is to help conclude abuse of all kinds, including racism.* When a trauma pattern lifts off for good, my clients and I have seen that what is revealed is not white, but rather clear, radiant, compassionate, healing essence. In this sense, the true opposite of black is not white, but *clear*.

So-called, self-styled "whites" may have appropriated (abducted?) benefits from the "purer" connotations intuited by the use of the label white. Yet few of us have had the strength, vision, or leadership to carry ourselves past the perpetrations of our own patterns of abuse to the realm of *clear*, though I intuit that brain offers up all such patterns not for the sake of abuse, but for healing. This "we are white (*i.e.,* good people)" strategy at best has seemed to curb the excesses of white perpetrations, urging the white toward more vigilance against his/her sadism and externalized self-hatred. Yet is it safe or wise to allow ourselves to be so delineated?

That these color vibrational conditions do not apply to skin color, or racial, ethnic characteristics has been stressed in colloquial terms: "It's not the color of your skin which is important." Often this homily is offered as a social and political strategy, and yet the dense narrative of racism persists, without the promise of how to dissolve or even identify the underlying pattern. Could we go to an invisible level to find its point of origin?

Could applying the insights about black and the traumatic mechanism help? Certainly studies of racism and personality have dwelled in this territory. What if the dissolution of racism as a defensive, narrative commentary upon trauma patterning for all people—black, white, and other—might be accomplished ultimately at energetic, not exclusively narrative levels? It is confounding how resistant patterning can be when approached only through narrative, without awareness of trauma's effect upon narrative.

Creative as it has been, I am not suggesting that there has been anything "conscious" about African-Americans naming themselves black, beyond the intuitive, even compassionate understanding of the linguistic traps which black and white polarizations syntactically render. Nor, because this energetic strategy has not been heretofore applied to discussions of racism, has it been part of the dialogue and of the strategies which might have been devised out of that dialogue.

The black that blacks name themselves is *not* the black of held energy which I have been discussing. But the parallels between approaching blacks and approaching the black of trauma seem to me interesting. When we face another, separate being, a vibrational platform of trust may evoke our trauma, causing us to seek difference in narrative, rather than deal with our own black. Coming toward another, we approach through color, but not the color of skin. The dialogue about racism might be not as much about color as about the structure of trauma.

Black and Violence: Another Digression

If our brain approaches what it identifies as its black, or continues to stumble over it, maybe ten times a second, only to have it neurochemically run away or be pushed away, an impossible and tragic bind is quickly and often terminally set in place at the energetic level. Subsequent narrative forms such as sin, original sin, double binds, disease, scapegoating, etc., can express this energetic movement surrounding a lack of movement, something the brain "fears" and perpetuates.

I believe violence might be viewed as our brain's attempt to rid itself of this conundrum, assuming that it must *intend*, where in fact, the best strategy appears to be to carefully *witness* and *allow* to dissolve. I have been fascinated, how, armed with guns, movie cowboys have a showdown which ends in fistfights, a *headbanging* strategy of brain, namely to punch out, or get someone else to dislodge, the unmanageable toxicity of trauma which the bad guy embodies. That such violence is itself a retraumatization, rather than a resolution of the patterning seems ironic in the extreme. And that violence shares this conundrum with other addictive processes is not a new insight, is it?

In Sophocles' *Oedipus Rex*, when Oedipus the King discovers that he has been unable to avoid the oracle's prophecy, and he has killed his father and married his mother, he puts out his eyes. The self-blinding narrative demonstrates the trauma mechanism, showing how the brain encodes in black the held-energy systems of traumatic experience, and then, as victim, proceeds to perpetrate it. And like our expulsion from the Garden of Eden, may be a retraumatizing narrative which does not describe the real trauma (see Chapter Seven).

The narrative of *Oedipus Rex* addresses dissociative process in us all and is plot-coded chronologically in reverse to invite resolution of the spectators' own dissociative process. In effect, the self-blinding of Oedipus is telling the traumatized brain how it got black in there, by its own protective mechanism. Oedipus wants to avoid the prophecy, yet he does perform the prophesied acts, under conditions of violence or stress which cannot be reexperienced directly or acknowledged by ordinary scanning brain. Narrative derived from our inability to penetrate held-energy black is doubly self-blinding.

The Oedipal black of Oedipus' self-imposed blindness is set in under conditions experienced as violent, and that it is, is part of the natural order of things. Suffering brain, it seems, has trouble figuring out why it cannot read the code. It is in Sophocles' *Oedipus at*

Colonus that we brains are shown how to resolve the held-energy patterning.

That Freudian psychoanalytic lineages often remained in the Oedipal narrative, rather than focusing on the black of the self-blinding, may have resulted in a hyperbolic retraumatizing of analysands like myself, who have struggled to align their personal narrative to Freud's commonplace developmental insight about parents and children. Hillman has argued similarly that psychoanalysis, as it has been, but perhaps is not now practiced, is an Oedipal process of self-discovery doomed to retraumatize, by its very analytic process.

The good news is that Freud's example of self-analysis has set us all returning to understanding ourselves as developing creatures who are, unaccountably, we think, stuck. Freud mobilizes the wave of exploration among others for whom the introspective life of classical traditions is not enactable. And by directing our meditational focus of awareness upon itself, initiates for so many the massive Western twentieth century movement toward individual and social healing.

Gray. One strategy is that grey is already different from black and may represent brain's attempt to detoxify or dilute the power of the black by placing white in juxtapostion with it. In that sense, gray might be considered a significant but a suspending phenomenon and my strategy has been to head again for the black. I treat gray like a pigment, so that within gray is black and white, and black can be abstracted from the gray by "zooming in" on a black sub-particle of the gray.

With experienced clients, I have attempted to see whether this magnification strategy is in fact sequential like a zoom lens, or whether there is a gap between the idea of zooming in and the "discovery" of the particle. Often people will hang out at the level of gray for some time before proceeding into the black.

Within some "liberal" political points of view, it is interesting how people who claim about reality that there are no blacks and whites, only grays, are arguing, perhaps rightly, against rigidity.

Using this strategy, within all grays, I find a hardcore black traumatic pattern which awaits dissolving. Might our conservatives' distrust of liberal talk reflect a narrative imitation of this energetic? The intuition is that liberal words belie the deeper immobilities. From the liberal point of view, conservative ideology unwittingly perpetrates the immobilities, retraumatizing at every point. Could both sides have it right?

Gray can also represent some more homogenized juxtaposition or assembly of black and white, than, say, alternating stripes, or mottling streaks, which also occur with regularity. Clients and I have watched how these transitional patterns have a rhythm or sequence which sometimes appears fixed but is not the bottom line of pattern resolution.

Silver. When the pattern shows silver, the black seems partially invested with movement but has not dissolved completely. Brain appears to move to *glossy surfaces*, implying as they can, a patinaed surface covering perhaps more difficult substructures. When we head into the black within the silver, a matte sub-surface often appears and, I think, places us deeper into the held-energy system. Sometimes silver almost conveys a reflecting surface and precedes the complexities of mirror vectors.

Orange. Orange tends to configure near deep black, or immediately after it; and as such, it seems to convey a beginning of transformation. It usually signals a status quo, in that with orange juxtaposed, the black appears in connection with something else, yet the basic traumatic pattern has not been resolved. In terms of trauma completion, I think orange is an early sign of movement, prior to and less complex than silver.

The appearance of orange and black at Halloween intuitively seems correct as an early invitation to trauma completion, though as we can surmise, all kinds of mischief can be perpetrated by patterns and systems which are only superficially resolved. In this sense, orange with black may be a temporary, potentially unstable respite

from deeper, more problematic, configurations, yet also a welcome
harbinger of movement and healing.

In a recent speech, one energetic researcher opined that orange
did not appear often in the body at an auric level. In fact, when
experienced from this perspective, not necessarily exclusively auric,
orange appears frequently.

Brown. When there is brown or darker shades of brown
initially trailing into black, like orange, it seems to reveal a transition
out of inert holding into energetic bruising. Here we are heading
toward healing resolution into a more organic configuration than if
we, like Henry IV at Canossa, are still kneeling in supplication in the
snow, as it were, outside the neurochemical gate of black.

With brown, we often go to the darkest part of the
configuration and watch what happens. I will ask a client what
direction to go in, toward the black or the brown. Sometimes the
black seems more manageable, sometimes the brown seems the first
order of business for brain. Once that has been resolved, the black
seems to reconfigure into something else, or some more manageable
shape.

When attributes of the brown change from repellant, bruised,
and obscure toward more organic forms, such as swamp, faeces, then
into ground, the tonus of the situation clears. When brown appears
as bark or refers to a tree, my intuition suggests we are in some
resolution of spinal or neurological trauma.

Tan, beige. Tan or beige can be approached as a variation on
brown, and can be divided into white or yellow and a darker brown,
as tonalities of gray can be resolved in a pointillist way into particles
of black and white.

Purple. Purple and its variants often appear associated with
powerful healing energy, hence its use for garments with magicians,
priests, and royalty. It seems to protect or to limit the power of a
held-energy system by appearing to corral or circumscribe the black

phenomenon. Other colors appear in this function, including yellow, white, green, and red. When approaching a multiple color configuration, we often head for the interface between colors, going toward the line between, say, purple and green, as a way of delineating the division and the unresolved energetic problem which appears to be puzzling brain.

It is possible to witness the colors as well as the black. Unless there is a mottled or special streaking, or repellant quality, "This is a color I have never liked," heading into the color rather than examining the boundaries and spacing between them becomes a judgment call which client and I share: "What do you think—where shall we go? What seems to be the next step?" Brain process will soon tell if the proper completion sequence has been found.

Just hanging out in the uncertainty will often promulgate some piece of the puzzle, setting it in its proper order, spatially and sequentially. At these sites, sequence itself can reveal the relationships between time and space in a way which strict plot or narrative only hints at.

Red. The connections which come with red can be traditionally associative ones, such as blood, passion, and inflammation. Sometimes entering the red will set off actual intensification of healing heat throughout some relevant, though rarely predictable part of the mindbody. With an awareness of the blood-brain barrier, some people are surprised by the realization that in terms of color, our brain itself is blood fed. Variations in the density and intensity of red seem to comment upon levels of completion.

Pink. Sometimes a harbinger of health, pink appears to report a change which the client often welcomes: "That feels better now, the area has a fleshy normal color to it." Again, in some configurations, there even seems to be some personality attachment to the color pink, and I have been intrigued by the ways in which the client initially will attempt to make the color, or shape, anatomically right.

When asked to describe their inner energetic landscape, clients will adopt what they know from anatomy or chemistry to get oriented. These views don't hold up very well in the long run. After a while, we can both feel how the artificiality of this attempt keeps us from energetic levels where change occurs.

Clients and I can usually tell when this kind of making up, or trying to respond to my suggestions to "please me" is in operation—brain lets us know when we are following its directions, not ours. The truer held-energy systems have a more abstract and fundamentalist reality than straight anatomy, though we often can drop into the vibrational levels from even those pictures.

Blue, green, yellow. These related colors will sometimes convey moods, as will other color groupings, or they will mix with black to create sickly colorings which repulse clients: "I have always hated this gray-green color," or "There's something wrong with this yellow-green." At their purest vibrational levels, they are enjoyed as some sign of progress which then takes the client to a levelling out place, "Something seems to have been completed," or "There's an infinite quality about this blue—like the sky," or to the next position of traumatic holding.

Gold. Gold is a wonderful vibration, for, as my colleague Wilhelm Heppe, knowledgeable in these esoterica, offers, it occurs when the personality, or that portion of it which conveys golden light, is in balance. While no one has yet reported a halo ring, I have had clients experience being bathed in radiant gold, being held in the hands of Christ or the Buddha, or hearing angels sounding heavenly golden horns near their ears as some energetic resolution occurs.

One friend for whom this happened asked me whether I too experienced the special energetic he and I had, as it were, manifest. "Was it as good for you as it was for me?" he joked. I intuited a higher vibrational state but did not directly experience the color/ vibration as gold. In sessions with clients, I act more as intuitive secretary and coach, though the changes at subtle energy levels are available to me some of the time, and I regularly comment upon them.

When we embody golden vibration, we are extensively relational, and our movement is characterized within what has been called the Golden Rule as well as the Golden Mean. Both rules acknowledge balance and proportion which I believe extends to, and in trauma is compromised, at the level of cellular memory. Heppe seemed impressed when I told him that clients were "getting gold" in our sessions, but, he reminded me, "That's not the bottom line. While gold suggests personality in balance, there is still some attachment to personality *per se* in the color."

I had sensed that, but was uncertain about the hierarchy, so I asked him, "What is the bottom line?" His answer, "No color—just clear." From this point of view, the appearance of all forms and colors reflect some attachment, and the goal of enlightenment can be phrased as the elimination of all illusion and suffering, where we can reside in clear. This can be a venue to the Tao.

At times I have intuited with clients that they try to witness the black, rather than get caught up in the perhaps premature comfort of the resolution which includes, say, vibration purple, or even gold.

Void. Void is void, not black. It has no density and has no shape, though clients have had interesting results focusing upon where some patch of void starts or ends. There is often a distinct boundary somewhere near or within void, usually a black line, like an horizon. When we enter void, it can be scary, and the dynamic of why the brain stays in the traumata rather than experience spacious void is, of course, a central issue.

Whereas trauma is coded in held-energy black, void has movement, or the potential for movement. It is like an empty canvas of space with no holding or prefiguration. The greater our tolerance for lack of traumata suggests we can exist at the energetic level where energy and void meet. Perhaps it is pretentious to suggest it, but I think we may be able to intuit something about beginnings of creation from that interface.

Forms

Square, cuboid forms suggest some rationalized function, but they are trappy, in that they appear attractive and ordered, whereas they are also rigid and held-energetic. When clear, our mindbody does not appear to have these structures, though energetically, like a *deus ex machina* of the Greek theater, or John Wayne and the cavalry, they seem to be evoked under stress to deal with traumatic impact. One way to approach these has been to ask the client, "From this point in the chemistry, what [does brain say] needs to be done?" We are always moving toward the point where brain does not know what to do with the form that appears.

Often, this is the first time this question has been posed in this portion of the chemistry. I think this question may be the most substantial form of intentionality in an approach which is designed to reduce intentionality to a minimum. Usually, the brain offers a number of approaches to these forms, including the following:

1. Nothing needs to happen.
2. It's fine, I guess.
3. What do you think should happen? Let me please you about this by asking your opinion or advice.
4. I don't like it, but what can I do?
5. I don't like it, and I can get it out by lifting (smashing, pulverizing, visualizing, etc.) it out.

None of these solutions ever satisfy, in part because any of the above solutions leave us with some sort of structure, even powderlike, which seem to clutter up, deviate, and clot clear energy movement. These sequences usually end up with the client determining by some crude logic that we cannot bang or smash these densities out, and that the form or color needs to self-transmute. Theologians and psychologists might talk here about surrender; then something else occurs.

Circles, spheres: These are variations of held energy in acceptable, coping function shapes. They have various surfaces, including shiny, and when they are shiny, they seem to have a glamorous, Hollywood quality. I feel better when the color turns to a dull black. That appears to signify that the surface has been addressed as surface, and somehow the surface is recognized (*anagnōrisis*) as insubstantial or somehow irrelevant; the shiny surface will peel away, leaving a more problematic under-layer ready to be addressed. Sometimes clients will hover in these partially resolved problem areas for days, weeks at a time.

Diamonds, faceted jewel, pyramid, and crystalline structures: I have had luck with the following approach. I recommend clients navigate the line where two planes or surfaces join. It seems to me our brain organizes a narrative of conjoined or abutting facets to "explain" vector shifts of energy, but because they have the fixed quality of a jewel shape, their density, in however attractive and alluring a form, is not flowing, is not clear. One can be drawn to possess the jewel rather than the clarity which is hiding even below this attractive, precious level.

Almaas describes diamond awareness, which, my guess is, must be ultimately dissolved. Likewise, pyramids or crystalline shapes convey a distinct stability which seems secure, but which ultimately will transform when the pivot point of origin of the relevant held-energy system is discovered. With these faceted structures, the task appears to be to experience the vector shift between adjacent planes.

One client, who had been in a bad accident five years before, had been working with a black pyramid for days. She noted red "blood" appeared to be pouring out a hole at the top and flowing down the sides. Asking "What needs to happen?" she reported that the blood flow needed to stop; it felt hemorrhageal. She focused down the hole to the base of the pyramid.

"What's down there?" I asked.

"A lot of vessels," she reported. I intuited this was not the direction to go in. We returned to the pyramid itself. "Can you get into the body of the pyramid just to witness its vectors? Go down the opening and face the tube wall and see if it can be entered at ninety degrees, such that you can come out the side angled surface of the pyramid."

"It can, but I get confused. There's too much to get lost in."

"Perhaps the same vector shift can be experienced higher up," I suggested. "Go down only a little bit from the top, and go out through the tube wall, to the sloping facet." The client was quiet.

"Wow," she exclaimed. "A large black column is rising out of the hole in the top of the pyramid. It is hovering. Now it's sweeping along the outer surfaces of the pyramid in sequence. Now it is gliding above the hole and is dropping back into it."

"What is happening to the black column?" I asked.

"It's melting down in the heat of the red. And there's no more red on the sides, and the pyramid is white."

"Are you intending any of this?" I asked.

"Nope," she replied, "it's just happening."

"How does that feel?" I asked.

"Better," she said.

Glossy and matte surfaces: With some clients, the presentation of glossy surface suggests that the underlining pattern will not be addressed, or cannot be because of its difficulty. Perhaps we are distracted by its reflective movement. At these moments, reminding clients how hard these tasks can be seems useful, because the nature of our energetic difficulty is so different from what we would ordinarily think is difficult. While glossy can also indicate some movement, matte seems closer to the center of the pattern.

Rough and smooth, corrugated surfaces: These, like glossy and matte, may tell us something about ways to approach the surface of a held-energy system so that it can be understood. I may suggest that the client scan into a groove, or along the surface, or "take a microscope" and go to a level of magnification where it starts to get more difficult. Focusing along the lines of vector of the density usually evokes changes.

Mirrors: Psychologically, the problems with mirrors are manifold. First are issues of reverse reflection. When looking in the mirror, left is the same side in the image as it is in the observer who is being reflected, not the case when we face another person. Also, we encounter left and right crossing over, witnessing ourself, narcissism, all deriving from or can be commentaries upon our experiences of mirrors. Yet the actual structures of mirrors include layers of glass, quicksilver, and black. And when we hang out with energetic mirrors, they do not act as mirrors in the sense of seeing our self in them.

Mirrors may report some chemical function which is reflective, refractive, perhaps encapsulated, and thus brain narrates this function using them to do so. I am not satisfied with my understanding of this aspect of the work, though I think it has something to do with more than witnessing oneself, either directly, or in dissociative distancing, such as when we experience leaving our bodies and watching what is happening to us.

Vectors

There are recognizable patterns which recur. In describing them energetically, I find myself using words like vector, torque, and skew. *Vector* seems to mean an energetic directionality or intentional line, while *torque* refers to a twist, or rotation often surrounding or affecting the spine or some limb. *Skew* means tilt or angle from an implied baseline, usually vertical, as in the spine.

The cross. One pattern sequence is when a vertical becomes horizontal, or vice versa. There is something here about the cross configuration which expresses orientation to gravity and of course carries loads of traditional symbolic values. By holding our attention to some place on a distinct vertical, the energy often reconfigures into an horizontal.

Sometimes the interface between horizontal and vertical is fused, sometimes it is separated, with one vector overlapping the other.   These are not inconsequential formulations, as they may represent brain's attempt to manage crisis, and certainly to reflect its power to perpetuate it.

What appears as a matter-of-fact cross, upon further examination may become a series of vectors which need to be allowed to pull out from the central crux. Crosses can be a set of four abutting right angles. One of the more difficult energy patterns to solve is the conjoining of the legs of a **right angle**. We take right angles for granted as an everyday reality, rather than an extraordinary assembly of radically juxtaposing vectors. We might argue that because of its particular vector difficulty, and in the face of its pervasive appearance, energetically speaking, the only angle is the right angle, for it characterizes all angles placed *in extremis*.

In the realm of energetics, the right angle appears decidedly different from our inner universe of curves, movement, and ultimately, clear space. When a rectilinear form occurs, I often suggest the client go to one of its right angles and focus upon one of the legs, then scan down the other, and experience the effort that juxtaposition entails. Often angles form arrowheads, and I suggest clients focus right at the position brain is pointing out with the angle. Often that focus will induce transformation of the form into **spheres, amoeboid forms, balloons, curvilinear "objects"** which suggest a new phase in brain's attempt to liberate itself from the rigidities and rationalizations of its held-energy systems.

In Chapter Nine, I speculate upon the representation of traumatic process which the figure of Jesus on the Cross entails. Here, I suggest that the soul, the gestalt of energy, may be affixed to its own rigidified image of itself. Incarnation is crucifixion. Another way to see it is our mindbody in trauma cannot achieve true horizontal and vertical balance, and enters, dies, into a held-energy system, leading to "ascension," a transformation and a self-dissolution of that system.

Some crosses need to be allowed to tease themselves apart. They seem energetically proposed in the traumatic moments to exist as held-energy outriggers. As such, they can represent an attempt to hold skewing forces under extreme duress to a viable image of balance, and for that reason their appearance means we are not at the bottom of the pattern. Christian theology suggests that all suffering can be gestalted into Jesus on the Cross, and that makes some sense, in that all traumatic patterning can configure into an image of pseudo-balance from which further "letting go" is possible.

Another related pattern involves **shifts from left to right**, and **right to left**. In the cases of physical trauma, such as falling off a ladder, the holding points appear to be on, say, the left, where the chronic pain appears. But by following the vector of the line—asking brain what needs to happen—the opposite side reveals itself as the locus of deeper stuckness.

Rolfers and other bodyworkers know this left/right so-called compensatory phenomenon, which resembles the protective male pheasant which distracts the hunter's attention away from the more vulnerable female and her chicks. Recent research at Yale documenting contra-lateral neurological pathways between left and right hemispheres might identify tissue levels of this energetic.

The left-right axis is not the same always as the horizontal, and depending upon the complexity of the patterning, can skew at places wherein it seems as if the body parts were placed under snapping pressures like a twig breaking across a knee. When a balance is achieved, the vertical and horizontal appear equalized in some way, and quickly disappear.

Another pattern is **top to bottom**. Reichians have long noted how held energy will close off whole segments of the body, sometimes with catastrophic results. They take the held energy literally and deal with it as a block. I have not observed Reichians use (color) vibration at the level I am discussing to evoke trauma resolution, and we can all get caught in the swamp of retraumatization, going over the pattern but not allowing it to resolve itself. But the Reichian lineage, now encompassing all mindbody work, more than other Western lineages I have encountered, has encouraged therapists to observe the energetic shifts and to honor them.

Spinning. There are times when a nebula-like pattern will begin to spin. Clients "hop a ride" on the spinning, depending upon the speed. If the pattern can slow down, then a change takes place. Sometimes this spinning is like a vertigo or dizziness. If it seems too much, clients usually focus upon our skin to skin contact between my fingers and the base of their head to ground the process. Sometimes I wonder whether this spinning is toxicity or something else. Often, these phenomena turn into funnels.

Funnels, whirlpools (tornadoes). Funnel-shaped phenomena appear within the energy sequences, and I have assumed they are or are like the chakra experiences reported by Barbara Brennan. Only they don't always "site" at the traditional loci of the chakras in the body. Could that be because they occur within dissociative toxicity? Are they reformulations of some pre-windshield chaos? Clients will report "going into and down" a vortex, and usually come out the other end with a resultant pervasive clarification of energy throughout our mindbody.

Craters and fissures. Often on the surface of a particle there will be craters or gatherings creating fissures. If we can focus upon the bottom of these, they yield a movement similar to the funnels. Often clients will express fear, then say that they are going toward the bottom anyway—the process is already unfolding, as if there is no real choice—then find an opening, through which a lightening of the pattern or complete revision occurs.

Caves, tubes, and tunnels. Surfaces are significant in that they appear to convey the neurochemistry of boundaries, and we can sense the difficulty of approaching and of penetrating them. In magnification, they show caves and declivities that lead into tube sequences, wherein a lightening is perceived at the end of the tunnel, as brain articulates an obscured chemistry. Often clients will render what appears to echo a birth while moving through these, though it is interesting to me that some do not make the obvious connection in their understanding; they seem to be immersed in the process.

When stuck in a tunnel, we often face the wall at a ninety-degree angle to its plane and the longitudinal axis of the tunnel. From there we can often focus into and through the wall, and bring brain to recognition of the wall's energetic nature.

Flat and three-dimensional forms. When the forms appear two-dimensional, I believe the pattern reflects greater dissociation. Movement around to the back of the system will clarify **front to back** differences, as well as the crucial point of transition between front and back. Along that line I think we often see some aspect of the spine. When the form becomes three-dimensional, as with characters in literature, we are moving into deeper levels of the held-energy system. This volumetric dimensionality shows up in personality as deepening, less shallow, more radiant affect.

Peeling and crumbling. When brain is beginning to reformulate its understanding of a certain process, the surface of the particle which has presented as problematic will start to peel or crumble. In spinal trauma, the energetic spine, or segment of spine, often will appear as a steel rod. As that is examined, the steel will be seen as a coating which will then peel, revealing a brown tree-like structure, bark-like, *i.e.*, more organic, then something more spine-like appears. Then, if one enters the brown as color, the energy is "released," and significant reformulations of torques and rotations are possible within a very short time. We wait and watch the process or realignment. Plastic forms can also peel away. Below, I comment more on plastic.

Plastic. Recently, a colleague was working on a pattern which increasingly seemed to pertain to a hysterectomy, and scanned as a white plastic shuttlecock lying horizontally in the field. We discussed the image, and then she went into one of the rectangles in the flanging plastic web of the shuttlecock. The space duplicated the angles of a previously occurring side-view portion of plywood—there, apparently, an image of spinal trauma and compression. In enlargement, the space became a column, and the viewing vector shifted ninety degrees, so the rectangular space approached horizontally, once entered, was now vertical.

The plastic column "became" flanged at top and bottom, like a breast pump, and filled with "milk." She directed her focus to the plastic, then to the "milk," which was getting thicker, then to the interface between milk and plastic. The energetic of the milk seemed to be toxic, and not organic, and we both thought it may have been the energetic of spinal anaesthetic, going back as far as the operation (eight years), perhaps much earlier into a lineage of pelvic and blood pressure disorders through three generations of women in her family.

The plastic then disappeared and the column became much thicker, yet somehow more manageable. It turned into a "safe" lollipop form, with a looping cord handle. We both thought that the brain had separated or held as a kind of energetic marker the "plastic" from the original (comforting?) anaesthetic mass, which was on some level indigestible and foreign.

Now that brain understood what it was, the plastic could disappear and merge with the white thick column fluid, and somehow now had found a way to neurochemically comprehend or begin to digest and presumably "excrete" the toxic energetic vibration. The cherry-red lollipop now was "blood-like" at its head, and the cerebrospinal system at this point in the chemistry appeared now characterized as a handle looping, moving up and down in two-way traffic, as it should.

We felt the entire session, as the previous one, had been cruising through spinal column trauma, and she had made some headway into a very complex set of chronic distortions, affecting her metabolism and sense of well-being. Instead of her earlier, presenting frantic, even mortal despair, after the session my colleague felt hopeful and connected, though the pattern was not fully resolved.

Here, plastic indicated something not organic, whereas in some sequences, brain uses it to convey an improvement, say from a steel immobilization energetic to something more manageable.

Exceptional colors and situations

When brain perseverates over an enchanting, dazzling pattern which evokes approach and avoidance movements, one question I ask is, "Is this a foreign substance?" Brain then can focus upon a particle to see what needs to happen. Usually, brain is overwhelmed by the sparking, spiking radiance, and does not perceive a). that the "particle" must leave the system, and b). how to get it out.

Under such focusing, one young man went into LSD flashbacks, which had disturbed him for a long while, not knowing that he could remove the chemistry from within. Another woman, alchemically, it seemed, transformed a natal anaesthetic into a root, something organic, and reported significant reduction of stress and renewed sense of space within her body. Recently, and increasingly, my practice has included successfully clients who wish to conclude addictive relationships established neonatally with caffeine, nicotine, alcohol, and other toxins.

CHAPTER FOUR: TECHNIQUE CONSIDERATIONS

Change

As a way of establishing a time frame for this approach, I have intuited that it would take only "twenty minutes" to revise most held-energy systems at the point of origin, but, as we say, they have to be the "right" twenty minutes. It might take me a year, or years, before I could line up my chemistry to support some final completion in the place where I am stuck. And it would take time afterward to integrate the new information throughout my personality database, particularly the loss of the old held-energy system.

Sometimes, clients and I can guess how far away from the center of the trauma they are, and I use the word *moment* to describe those intuitions: "I think you are moments away from concluding the pattern."

"How long will that take in real time?" the client asks.

"Can't say. Maybe two minutes, two weeks, two months, two years. But as observing coach, outside your process, it seems to me you may be only a few steps away." Or "It may take some getting used to the toxicity of the system you are working with, but if you go at it slowly a bit each day, you can reduce the scale of the system."

Sometimes I get bogged down in the details and spatial relationships being described, and it can be easier to work with paper and pencil to communicate, particularly in settings where touch is forbidden. I have worked next to clients in some cases, or across a room, or facing them at a desk with pencil and paper. There can be a mutual strategizing between client and practitioner to see what works. To go into prenatal material, to scan the deepest trauma patterning. my intuition is that clients should be held and held uninterruptedly throughout the session.

I remind clients that if they can bring their "primitive" brain to look at the pattern, they may not need to understand it or relive it in the old way of reenduring the original trauma as happened in the movies *Equus*, and *Suddenly, Last Summer*, even though I have done some of that, as described in my stepping on the glass fragment.

We rightly fear the immobilities expressed through the narrative level, which appear thus correctly, overtly revealed, and irremediable. To ascend from these crucifixions involves more dedication than people initially have. We just want the pain and suffering to go away.

Clients may experience aspects of their trauma and have insights which would make an analyst drool, but these seem less significant to the vertical movement into the black of the held-energy system, and hence into change. Interacting with the held-energy system at an energetic, not a narrative level, seems to allow the client to witness trauma completion at a less cluttered, more direct level.

From this perspective, asking a client to reengage at the narrative level can be retraumatizing to start with. It may be more approximal luck than anything else when our held-energy systems are resolved within the rubric of these (psychodynamic) narrative reenactments. We thus may not focus on the learning that needs to take place if the pattern is to be detoxified and dissolved. In that sense traumatic resolution occurs in an *educational* context, where the information is finally processed in the proper order which brain determines, at the proper level and density where brain has it stored.

How can we know change has occurred? We can tell somewhat by the degree of stress that drops away even in the session. Clients will notice afterward how the troughs, nooks, and crannies which subtly would preoccupy or carry them in some direction are now lightly filled-in, as unaccountable sources of energy and support instead of depletions. They have an airy quality, and new patterns and inner avenues or vistas become supportable and supported.

Thought patterns, addictions, no longer dominate Often they disappear quickly and permanently, the way we have always dreamed they would. Often the change is quite dramatic, where a spinal rotation or neck torque pattern will dissolve as our cellular mind/body sets itself again in motion.

Completion

If a black system slides off-stage, or off the scan of our awareness, or it disappears radically as we are trying to fix on it like spearing an unruly *hors d'oeuvres*, then it seems it will return. If it dissolves, or crumbles, and melts down in front of us, the pattern is reconfiguring, and it appears to be no longer a problem at that level. Brain often acknowledges when fragments remain and when the pattern seems to be concluded, and the client will report it as such: "Something seems to have been completed here."

When there are stages or sequences to a greater held-energy system, the problem of witnessing it seems more complex. Levine has noted how traumata "stack" or spindle, one on the other. Narrative debris may tell you how the brain has organized its response to many and repeated patterns. After scanning these various settings, moving into the energetic through color will usually reduce the broth to its essential movement, perhaps taking us as far back as birth, or farther.

Our brain may reveal how the initial scatter occurs, but in order to gather the parts into the same framework for observation of their relationships, we may have to go from place to place—the twitch in the leg, the pain in the neck, the dark patch at the base of the spine. Most "places" are fragments, like post-big-bang planets, from which entire universes can be observed. In a holographic sense, I intuit there is only one pattern that needs to be learned in any one place, but that possibly reflects a higher level of trauma resolution than our dissociation initially allows.

Using this strategy, all patterns are problems, and even those we like keep us at a distance from (the) energetic, and its ultimate, (the) clear.

Focusing

I have discovered that the only level of intentionality that can be applied in this energetic work, if anything, is that of focus. And that should be done without predetermination of what should be seen. Within this rubric, and like many other techniques constructed around the same intuition, bringing intention would be retraumatizing. *We follow the directions on the package*, the order in which brain wants to or can resolve its own chemical and energetic understanding.

It seems to me classical therapists offering their stock interpretations ("You hated your mother") are in consistent violation of this intuition and, from this point of view, risk retraumatizing on a wide scale. If this is true, no wonder some analyses have been endless, and, if the reports of some analysts are to be believed, at some critical point, deemed unsuccessful. Of course, they are not unsuccessful. Merely the bottom of the pattern has not been reached.

The basic underlying patterns that organize experience, that are noticeable and are not blended into awareness, appear to the owner personality and to others as behaviors, tendencies, predispositions, characteristics, and personalities. I observe that these patterns are subject first to the rules of held-energy systems at a preverbal, energetic level. This energetic level is so far from our usual, traumatized and retraumatizing awareness which we ordinarily experience as ordinary, that to enter this level might seem initially to court insanity. But all great systems of healing, recognition, and enlightenment are based upon recognition of its factual nature.

Within this rubric, returns to language and the language centers of the brain essentially may be retraumatizing by their very nature, as may be employing will and intention. These patterns are the ones upon which all subsequent patterns spindle, because they are the oldest, first ones that the brain refers to for guidance as to how to get through any crisis. Colloquially, we may return to the neurochemistry trackings of our relatively successful beginnings, such as birth, every time we face a new situation.

The most important patterns that organize our experience seem to me preverbal, prenatal, genetic, intuited, energetic, or part of karmic "former life" directionalities, hence are beyond words. So the use of words upon these patterns can be an obvious intrusion. I have come to think that at the deepest level, only the traumatized brain can heal itself, with only the practitioner's energetic platform support. At these critical points our brain will not tolerate any crossing of boundaries by will or intention, as, say, in some modalities. Anything less or more does not seem to allow the held-energy system to self-dissolve.

Furthermore, the use of language between client and practitioner can convey direction and where to focus, but ultimately, our brain wants to experience completion, whether in the often necessary company of another person or "alone." This reorganization requires its own neurochemical firing, at a level of complexity that defies commonplace intervention. Clients and I note how the patterns complete in ways which neither one of us would have ever guessed or could have intuitively implemented.

What some clients and friends suggest as a way to make this technique-approach user friendly is to frame it as a form of *conjoint meditation*. Certainly it borrows from meditative strategies and lineages, though I have never experienced guidance toward focus of this direct type in any of the mediational practices I have been exposed to, though often I have wanted something like this.

In addition to meditational antecedents, I think this technique accompanies the same insights that garner impressionism and symbolist poetry of the nineteenth century, though I have revaluated that only recently. Like all techniques, however, this one has developed out of my own necessities for efficacy and understanding as client and as practitioner with clients.

Specific Strategies for Addressing Energy Configurations

Here are some strategies clients and I have developed.

When there are lines, head for the lines. Or the outlines. When there is a hiatus—the pattern gets lost, or moves abruptly—see if it can be regained. Go to the body part or the original place sensed and get it back as you trace the pattern again from where it first showed its (a) face.

Return to the early images to ask how they look. Evaluate how much they have changed, or what has happened in the meantime. Both client and I usually find that interesting.

Wherever there is black, head for it. Try to get it decoded by dividing it into smaller and more basic units until the whole system dissolves. The colors surrounding the black may be important. Sometimes they seem to hold, contain, or limit the (toxic) trauma capsule, as it were, and while the vivid colors seem preferable or more attractive, in those cases we can support brain's staying with the black.

I refer the insights and memories that come up when the black is entered to the (figurative) drying rack behind me and the client—we are, I explain, like potters throwing pots—or to similarly located "archives," for future retrieval if needed. Likewise, all insight, prejudice, and disbelief modes of thought can be suspended in the archives while brain is escorted into the energetic.

Where colors interface, or are blended, those interfaces and the boundaries implied are important, and often a black line or cross will emerge to show some shift in chemical vector. Then the black can be "entered." Sometimes, the background will be a true background, not directly connected to the foreground particle within view.

We often go to the interface of the boundaries. Wherever there are boundaries, that indicates some kind of truncation of the energy. When the energy is flowing, it is self-regulating, and presents as a balanced golden radiance, cusping into clear, and does not need external boundaries. Or internal ones. In that neurochemistry, it does not "make errors" of judgment or move out of impulse or ignorance.

We can argue that free will is what we experience when we are energetically flowing clear. We have choice beyond ordinary choice, farther and deeper, and perhaps more frighteningly spacious than we are accustomed to characterize it. For the remainder of our experience, in traumatic process, we are in the tyranny of a determinism, not so much of the ordinary kind, but of a set of determining held-energy patterns we cannot even see, nor are we allowed to until we set out toward being clear. Our traditional juxtapositions of free will and determinism are important for they can illuminate not a true contrast of essences, but of phases of traumatic process.

Breath and Oxygen Processing

There is a cellular clarity which then can be witnessed as linked to our *breath*, but my experience so far is that that connection should not be obscured or anticipated by breathing technique. For those like myself, some breathing functions seem to be located at or within held-energy patterning. Trauma at birth and after can take our breath away. Thus, when breath is linked to held-energy systems, it is difficult for us ever to experience the radiance that emerges when we are clear.

Whatever split that occurs between oxygen processing and traumatic holding requires that we sometimes get caught in layering, manifest here spatially as one layer separated from another. So that there are held-energy systems, plus layers within those, plus the trauma mechanism itself to deal with.

Our brain does not understand its own bureaucracy of protection, plus the activation of that system, which is something else. In short, lineages of breathing exercises like those in yoga may duplicate their historical development or discovery, *i.e.*, from the held-energy systems within each individual who discovers this or that way of breathing.

Significantly, clients integrating the breathing chemistry sequence of say, Boston, 1995 with the trauma time of say an accident in Shreveport, 1945 often experience a sense of suffocation and of not being able to breathe. This is scary and often very uncomfortable, but with guidance, the interface as the older (non-)time is connected with the new, present time can be managed.

If clients ask me what can they do by way of homework between sessions, I encourage them to reside in their own breath and notice what happens within. I report my own progress watching my breath patterns. Currently, when working alone on my patterns in the early waking minutes of the morning, I focus upon where the breath and oxygen processing is blocked or compromised.

What Happens?

What happens when the client can't find the pattern or any pattern? So far, I have not experienced that. Patterns can be momentarily lost, or their initial appearance is not obvious, but with time, they declare themselves. When a pattern begins to dissolve, there is a sense of completion, sometimes with radiant, golden energy coursing through the mindbody.

What happens when there is a process or movement going on? I suggest to the client ahead of time that they should wave me off in some fashion, indicating they are in some process or they are scanning. I then shall assume it is too complex, or preverbal, or too fast to give it words, and that our talking would interfere in the process. Later, they can tell me when some process has completed, or they get stuck.

What if clients cannot see in this new way, or they can only sensate? There are many entry points into the energetic, but individuals may have trouble accepting the vibrational as real, or significant. Even with results, they will deny its place. Meditators or those familiar with art, yoga, high-level sports, or martial arts have less trouble than some others, which may say something about preparation for letting go of form and hanging out in formlessness without getting scared. All of this can be approached playfully and respectfully.

So far, the negotiations have been generally quite informal and playful, with lots of strategizing about where the best place is to go, what the difficulties are, etc. At times the specificity of the work, and the focus involved make our sessions seem like surgery. And clients report feeling they have been through a real workout, experiencing fatigue of an unusual sort at the end of sessions. We have found drinking pure water and rest helpful.

What happens when the client cannot follow our, their and my, directions to a proposed viewing place? At times I will say, "I don't know where to go from here," or "What needs to happen here? What does brain want?"

The strategies can become quite literal: "Try viewing it from another perspective—back, side, whatever." Usually that will gain us entry to a new phase of the problem.

Apparent capacities of the self-examining brain

Here are some further ideas.

I find it is useful to acknowledge that our brain appears to be able to focus upon its experience at any number of levels of magnification. Like a camera, or a spaceship, it can zoom in and out, view microscopically or in broader overview, can compare positions, and can describe what it sees. I have been curious to hear from clients how the spatial language which emerges when people are describing their inner energetic workings are often completely disavowed by so-called professional therapists as not possible, nor relevant, nor true.

The sensations of our brain, with perhaps the notable and sad examples of headaches, are often denied, or thought to be signs of emotional disorder, and the attempt to acknowledge such is rejected within some traditional medicine lineages. Clients will complain to me of condescension and reinterpretation on the part of their therapists, who judge and politicize their encounters, rather than probe the reality from within the system-pattern as it appears.

These therapists seem to try to set the pattern within a frame of meaning, symbolic or otherwise, pulling us back into the language and symbolic centers of the brain, as if these have the ultimate claim to our allegiance. Their symbols can be retraumatizative in nature, built upon insight and linguistic structures proposed by the brain, not the energy itself, all of which forms are "symbolic." By whose authority is this "therapeutic" positioning allowed, or even more haplessly, certified?

Our brain appears to be able to move around held-energy configurations, go behind formulations of its own making, attend to vectoral shifts when they occur, such as in diamond or rectangular shapes ("Go to the point where the three sides of the cube meet.").

Formulations of structure which the scanning brain can "witness" may be viewed ultimately as configurations of energy density. But the emotions and the narratives which accompany them seem untrustworthy as the bottom line, for the basic patterns which are laid in either in so-called former lives or our current neonatal experience, appear to act as primary spindle for subsequent traumatic experiences. That makes sense because in the speed or power of the traumatizing occasion, brain and its chemistry will revert to or invoke its earliest, most successful transaction under similar life-threatening conditions.

If we want the deepest change, the deepest freedom and clarity, I think we must lead our mindbody beyond narrative, beyond form, to the earliest realms of pure energetic. I think it is from this point that the best relationship of emotion and denser forms of incarnation can be dynamically observed and completed.

Holographic scaling

The brain has a rapid, computer-like function, such that once a new freedom has been discovered, brain recomputes, and new insights, cast up like Hansel and Gretel's breadcrumbs, show the trail of that energetic reworking.   No matter how overwhelming the pattern initially appears to be, it can be reduced to some manageable particle level in number and in scale.

We notice that patterns seem to be held cellularly throughout the system, each in the vectors skewed to the traumatic impact of the original experience.   It is as if all the cells in the pattern have their right front bumpers similarly dented, though this denting might be molecular, or neurochemical, not just grossly structural. Brain seems to work extrapolationally and holographically, in that if we attend to one segment of the picture, and "solve" it, brain generalizes from the specific.

We do not have to focus upon every cell or molecule. When one particle changes, entire archipelagoes of systemic, linking cells or molecular configurations of stress and alignment in our mindbody complex transform. Clients report sensing them reworking in the form of energetic waves, heat, even entire muscular, postural chronic stress reductions.   How far advanced stages of deterioration could be reversed in the held-energetic systems of, say, cancerous process, is a question I am just beginning to explore.

Stress can be viewed as resulting from unresolved trauma and the attempts (unsuccessful) of brain to resolve or complete the traumatically held actions or movements. So-called conscious, *i.e.*, dissociated, thought centers do not have to "understand" in the way of garnering insight, but brain seems to have to apprehend if there is to be change. It also will show it has understood by the insights it throws up to awareness.

For this reason, I remind clients that insight should not be considered the same as movement. It may be useful to strategize that insight reflects and comes after energetic movement. In that sense, insights are signs along the highway, telling us where we are, but they are not the highway, nor our movement on it.

Concomitantly, when plural forms appear, such as ones suggesting trees in a forest, one strategy is to assume that we are witnessing the effect of a post-big-bang shatter effect, often running parallel to the spine. If we stay with the detailing of the one entity brain finds most interesting (here, tree), the patterns usually resolve into one major tree, which then rescales and resolves into some deeper black pattern before completing into healthy, earthy brown and then clear. In a similar rendering, Odysseus/Telemachus slay Penelope's plural suitors and the singular Odysseus finally is reunited with his wife.

The spine and its traumata form a major piece of the action, and the images, rods, pipes, strings, tubes, etc. in the later stages of healing turn from hard metallic to plastic, to vegetative brown, tree-like, then to flesh-like, then into surges of energy which move serpent-like up and down the spine. These surges are recognizable to those who work with kundalini, yoga, high-level sports, and the martial arts. We can witness the vectors of the original impact by how far from the vertical the pipe, or tree, or branch lies. Often there will be more than one layer of skewed energy, set at differing angles to the vertical.

The scale of problems can be changed, even eliminated, dissolved. Like Alice in Wonderland, our brain suddenly shrinks or expands the patterns or forms. When the form shrinks, it seems as if the hyperbolic immanence of our traumatic chemistry is being reduced to appropriate proportion: "This is not as big a problem as I thought." When the forms get larger, I believe brain is closer to the center of the (exaggeration) scale of the original trauma's impact in and upon our chemistry.

But the information needs to be decoded first, not rationally nor analytically understood. That will come later and is evidence that the chemistry has changed. I find it best to ask clients to divide the massing of color into its component parts, for example, finding black and white in gray. This pointillist technique can then allow primitive brain to work on one portion of the problem.

With these changes in scale, I have suggested clients try to keep the pattern in focus by following and magnifying or changing perspective with the goal of observing the held energy at close range.

Sometimes this means zooming in on the energy as the form of the system reduces in size.

I recommend clients tell me what they are sensing as well as they can, though if they are in the middle of a process, not to talk and generally not to move, if movement is made to discharge the difficulty of the pattern. They give me signals, or at best freely ignore my requests for information.

This style gets to be quite comfortable between us, as if we are on a joint spelunking or scuba dive, and we have to figure out where to go next. The etiquette of the brain seems not unlike that of any new occasion: Where shall we go next? What seems to need to happen here? From this position, what needs to happen? How shall we evoke, or better, watch this change?

Intention and Retraumatization

From the perspective I am suggesting, energy is not considered overtly transferred or channelled between client and practitioner. In comparison to other healing modalities, I believe this is an important alternative when it comes, crucially, to intentionality.

If we intend colors, or images, such as "Send blue light into the place where it hurts," "Imagine the most beautiful place you have known, then find a Chinese philosopher and meet him there," etc., are we following the directions on the package?

If we place overlays of intention, positive thinking, imagery and the like, the patterns may temporarily change, and that may be positive for the client to know s/he can experience relief from horrendous patterns. But my experience is our root patterns do not transform with intention. At least the ones people come to me to help them complete and the ones which personally bother me. The accommodations most people make seem to be of the sort that they hold on to the basic stuck patterns and take relief measures in the form of temporary "releases," like repeatedly going to confession with the same sin, but never changing the basic premises upon which the sin is "structured."

The next phase is to allow that completion of the halted movement of the energy, momentarily and over time. I believe there is a growing body of practitioners who are working around ideas and theories like these, some not landing on the conviction that the brain can heal itself, because we take the narrative of immobility at "face" value.

With the support of another energy system, this waiting game appears to be the only acceptable, workable manner when the pattern appears intractable. It's a little like brain saying, "This pattern was installed under conditions of isolation, and I must return to that aloneness in order to re-solve its conundrum." Yet with the signficiant exceptions of witnessing and being in the presence of another energy system.

In situations where I make mistakes, including the usual one where I lapse into my own variation of interpretation, my error is in trying to intervene in the energetic process. For this kind of work, I have discovered that at the center of a held-energy system, brain (energy) must discover its own way through, and cannot be infringed upon.

Thus, from this perspective, every externally proposed, so-called visualization is a retraumatization. Every guided imagery is retraumatization, every willful or intentional intervention is retraumatization, whether it be by the brain of the practitioner-holder or of the client. In this, my understanding can approximate more the non-interventionist Christian Science position, though even Christian Scientists invoke the healing power of Jesus Christ, which in some applications may involve retraumatization.

My sense is that the Christ Scientist intervention may remove the full trauma, but might keep the client in a compromised sense of where the difficulty, and the authority lies (see Chapters 7-9). Christ energy, as I now witness it, lies both without and within the client, and certainly can be accessed relatively easily, given the permutations of trauma which the brain ordinarily tries to circumlocate in daily moment-by-moment experience as well as in attempts to heal itself.

I have used prayer occasionally for guidance and have shared that with the client as a strategy, though only as a way of delineating a non-interventionist position, for the client and for me. This neurochemistry has been advanced through the classic formulation: "Thy Will, not my will, be done." That we identify God's Movement with something as dense and traumatically determined as our so-called will might seem some height of humanoid grandiosity.

Judgment can be exercised by client and holder, and sometimes the voice of the holder-practitioner can be an interference, and so can the commentary. Any "interpretation" is offered as a strategy, not as the final place of understanding, which I take to be beyond narrative, beyond language itself. Such commentaries are a side-order of French-fries, not the main *entrée*. They are something to be noted and preserved in the "archives" as pivots into the next level, and, of course, eventually dropped.

I find that any total immersion into a held-energy system from the analytic level is not where mindbody ultimately wants to be. And the watchwords of this meditational, non-verbal bias are *Read the directions on the package*. The order of patterning which brain offers is the order in which the information of and within the held-energy system can be traced. Like Theseus emerging from the Labyrinth, we follow the string which we brains have set out.

The energy of the practitioner-holder is not channelled with intention, as it is in some aspects of Jin-shin, polarity, Reiki, or Rolfing, cranial-sacral, or healing touch modalities, for example. Both client and holder provide a neurochemical matrix of reciprocally relational energy which allows the client's primitive brain to offer up its held-energy system for mobilization and resolution, thus for self-healing. The practitioner's energy field can merely support and dovetail, running parallel to, coming up under, as it were, to match the ragged, uneven edges of the client's etheric patterns until by interfacing, itself a high vibrational state, the client's energy process can restore itself to balance and evenness.

Any further intentionality, implying crossing the (any) border, is again retraumatizing. Given a direct and consistent platform of energetic interfacing with another energy system, our brain will address whatever traumatic patterns most concern it. Client and practitioner merely have to witness, focus, and watch what happens next.

Interestingly, my experience with clients is that we float together in a matrix of energy which is mergy, but also boundaried. We can at times come back in our awareness to the place of skin to skin contact at my hands and their neck to check out the safety of this trust platform. If this platform is established, the client can move to what appear to be preverbal, prenatal, even pre-conception places quickly and with relative, increasingly playful ease.

At certain points in the process, I can remind clients that I think I am "running parallel" to their energy, not intruding upon it or intending into it. And that I am trying to stay out of my own hair as well. Our joint hope is that primitive brain will discover its own healing process and resources, usually from the darkest, most unassailable places, because we identify, focus upon, and witness those places.

Important problems of how to communicate the nonverbal occur at these points, and vocabularies of some complexity are proposed, set on the shelf, and we move on again into the shapes and color. I will comment out loud upon shifts which I sense ("Something has shifted."). Often these comments are "accurate" as to depth of connection between us and depth into the held-energy system we have achieved.

My sensations can be surprisingly congruent with the client's, and of course suggest that there is informational exchange between us beyond consciousness. But we try to let that be, rather than take control of it.

When rapport is established, the client can accurately report when they may be responding to my suggestions or questions, trying to please me. We usually then return to an earlier place and try going through the croquet wicket again from the proper direction.

Transference and The Unconscious

While pronouncedly *meditational,* my approach to these areas is matter-of-fact and playful, with opportunities for casual, humorous asides, puns, mistakes of direction—all of this kind of playful, even laughing exchange has been reported by non-touching analysts. What has not been as well reported nor experienced, is the *secondary* importance of the so-called transferential situation, which I think is based upon an inappropriate retraumatizing bonding, not upon the fact of touch itself.

When there is no possibility of touch at this level, with its implied responsive energetic interface, then, I think, a toxic transference may occur. The pattern is offered up and projected onto the therapist. The mutuality of the interface is obscured often by a pattern in the therapist's understanding which interprets the energetic as sexual, which in a professional setting is explicitly forbidden, hence no touching.

When there is the possibility of holding touch, a true parallelling function of the holder can occur, and there is no cause for lack of satisfaction, nor for projection, nor transference, nor counter-transference. These latter experiences are beside the point, not the point, as they are in traditional psychoanalytically-biased dynamic therapies. Brain has its own work to do. (How this apposite approach could be combined with non-touch by traditional modalities is something a few colleagues are exploring.)

Nor does there seem to be cause for the related concept of the so-called *unconscious* as an entity. The split which the concept of transference suggests may be a function of the dissociate mechanism of trauma, and certainly continually occurs, but does it appear to exist in a matrix of client-practitioner holding, separate from trauma function?

I have always been intrigued by the analytic texts which at the end of the discussion of the unconscious, treated as an entity, as in "Oh, that is my unconscious," indicate that there are some in the know who think there is no unconscious. As I initially perceived this idea it

seemed to me that such a conviction was an unenlightened, minority
opposition viewpoint. To say there is no unconscious did not
acknowledge the common-sense awareness which is that I often
perform activities in a dissociated state. At some level, I do not know
what I am doing.

But being in a dissociated state as I would now say it, is not
the same as viewing a construct as if it were always there, or had its
own mechanistic structure that could be discerned and evaluated,
particularly from an administrative overview of "The Unconscious: Its
Structure and Function." The concept of the unconscious may be
perhaps the strongest conceptual obstacle against entering energetic
realms which has been (self-)perpetrated in the culture recently,
always in the name of enlightenment.

Where the construct of an Unconscious applies may be in the
brain's recognition of the trauma mechanism, which produces held-
energy systems which the brain reads as solid and impenetrable. But
I believe these densities are not prior to traumatic processes. Yet
instead of proposing an unconscious, I am perhaps substituting the
idea of a consistent trauma mechanism.

People might ask, "But is there ever a time when traumatic
process is not being communicated, directly or indirectly, in the form
of character, personality, social influences, birth, bicycle accidents and
the like?" My reply is, "Probably not." As with the formulation of
Eden, the importance of envisioning a pre-trauma baseline is to reveal
the magnitude and ease of the problem of taking the patterns out and
living free of them. At the end of his life, absorbed in cancerous
process, Freud, for example, apparently could barely envision such a
sustainable state. Reich, on another hand, directly and often
commented upon the difficulty of sustaining the ecstatic.

My ordinary (it)-awareness of *the unconscious* has not been
particularly useful to understanding the trauma mechanism or
function, even though I know the lineage of its useage traverses the
same slopes I and my clients now also do. I tend to use the word and
the concept as a linguistic, analytic rescue station or float, when I am
heading into the sinking, or elevating sensation, partaking with subtle

energy. In short, the concept of an unconscious may be like a superstition, though the phenomena which cluster around its usage and which it tries to describe certainly are not.

In a dissociated neurochemistry, a state promulgated by our trauma mechanism, there is a residual if hidden energetic state which can be decoded and evoked, where the energy is cellularly vibrant and streaming. Reich, Whitman, and Blake, among others, identified and exalted that phenomenon. That revisionary, ecstatic objective does not translate into the usual conscious/unconscious grid as we talk about it, because consciousness usually means aware. Yet I think that what we are aware of is limited to our traumatic patterns, not the streaming where there is no ego nor held-energy systems to interfere or cause gravitational pulls upon otherwise free movement.

The particular manifestations in holding patterns and disease appear manifold and often predictable, but they have multiple permutations, endless, as from this perspective I see them, and diagnosis which does not recognize held-energy systems as (perhaps the primary) instigator may end up chasing its tail. If we follow the expert cancer doctors through a series of endgame maneuvers with a terminal patient, we can see the solipsistic patterns endured and perpetuated, and, with miracles excepted, morphine cocktails and death the only way out.

Changing the Trauma Mechanism

The trauma mechanism, with its potential for generating the tyranny and rigidity of long-term held-energy systems, perhaps cannot be changed. And what situations would we want to enter without its protective function at the ready? Yet the particulate manifestations of trauma which are reflected in obsession, fantasy, most sexual experiences, thoughts, longings, all seem so real that to consider them illusions in most cases appears to violate our sense of what makes incarnate life essential to our soul development. To challenge these assumptions for what they are, as "illusory," has been the task of regular life experiencers through the ages.

If I have a forbidden fantasy, or some pattern which has a torquey bit of kinkiness in it, I know that within even that formalized (decadent) structure, there is life force playing through, probably not directly and cleanly, but still playing through. To envision taking the pattern out, by repression, or by ignoring it, does a disservice to our mindbody, for it suppresses the brain's natural objective to be healed.

To play with details of the scanned pattern, such as with s/m variations, by acting them out, or analyzing them, may provide some sense of movement, but to hang out at that level for very long may perpetuate suffering. In fact, hanging out in that way may cause suffering, for it seeks to redress the imbalance without finding the source of the pattern, an old Buddhist insight.

Why has it taken so long for me to discover that the patterns are not perpetrated at the level which I think is awareness, nor that the patterns I think crucial are even relevant? In that sense to get caught in the so-called adjudication of these patterns where change is desired exclusively through morality or legislation seems to me to put the cart before the horse.

It has taken me a long time to fathom how when there is repetition, there is immobilization, and the immobilization is at a neurochemical, molecular level. When I focus appropriately at the vibrational level, here on color, the pattern will transform, be transformed, in the twinkling of some inner eye. The cognitive, behavioral, and insight aftermath of this energetic, even alchemical transformation is not known prior to it. The interest in transformation which usually brings people to this kind of work, remains to be rewarded and experienced.

I have seen this truth about the mechanism of trauma in many ways, on many levels, but in the place of my own trauma, I never see it. Its functioning is hidden from and by primitive brain. For me, the effective way to resolve these conundra now is with vibration, here again, specifically shape and color. I sometimes witness the color manifest at what must be molecular, or cellular densities, sometimes as a wave.

Increasingly I seek to experience myself at the level of a wave, rather than at the level of resolution of, say, a particle, or more substantially, a tissue, or muscle, or an assembly called mindbody. This approach gives me a more real sense of what I can be than if I am stuck at the original objectifying level, where the basic patterns appear stored.

My friend Mark Hochwender, an energy practitioner and therapist, reminds me that of course there are other vibrational levels with which to approach this clearing process, including smell, and significantly, sound. The latter he regards as ultimate, and there are times when I with my clients have experienced the interface between color and sound. What I use now is what I have needed to learn, and that is what I am sharing with you, friend-reader, here.

Hillman notes how the *Oedipus at Colonus* relies on sound for its more delicate surrender into transformation rather than the earlier, more sight-oriented *Oedipus Tyrannus* [*Rex*]. Yet it is very difficult to approximate the silence of held-energy, whereas absence of movement expressed visually by black may seem easier to access. And with more than one client, "seeing" the colors involves a different kind of intuitive seeing than they are used to when using their eyes. With more than a few, this can be a significant hurdle, usually overcome by asking them to sense, not see.

Dissolution of Patterns

In the moves I work with, the denser particles of black held-energy are dissolved into waves, into color. When I ask the client, "What does brain say needs to happen with this structure?" there are a number of usual responses: "I want to punch it out," "Let's shove this thing away," and "This doesn't belong here," are some of them. Then there is the classical working through, where brain finally realizes that it cannot even pulverize the denser energetics without some unresolved debris. Clear homeostasis implies a social, political, and economic energetic free of residue.

So the final answer seems to be, "It needs to be broken down, dissolved." It is my understanding that when we are at the origin of the traumatic pattern, structurally, or in time, dissolution (self-dissolution) is what happens. When the abstract scanned system slides away, or disappears quickly, or cannot be found, then my sense is that the pattern has not been completed. Brain knows and conveys when it has completed a problem.

That insight parallels developmental and psychodynamic insight, namely that if we are in rebellion, or push aside the pattern, then it comes back until we face the impossibility of the task. Then, as Aquinas acknowledges in the formulations of his *Summa Theologica*, the Godhead intervenes.

What does it feel like to lift off a pattern which we have not seen as a pattern, using color and vibration, rather than so-called insight understanding? From the place of restored balance, there can be a backward glance at the earlier phenomenon with the sense that now it does not belong (see Chapter 5, Session, lines 850-869).

Also, it may be interesting to ask if this new configuration is new information. After a while clients will be able to sense when it is and when it is not. Yet instead of the usual preoccupations and fantasies, obsessions, and the like of the rag and bones shop of our heart, there is a flow of energy which has a cellularly open quality and an absence of preoccupation.

We are able to enter and sustain fluidity, rather than the thoughts that fill and dominate our so-called empty space. Void is approachable. Why is it important to approach void? Like an existential flossing, by establishing a neurochemistry of clear, we broaden our vision of our limits, providing real, significant contrast to what we think we are and could be. Thakar notes that when we hover in the solitude, which is not void but has been confused with it, we can discover a vibrant and relational energy which transforms our connection with the world and with reality.

CHAPTER FIVE: FURTHER
STRATEGIES AND ANECDOTES

Getting Out of the Way: Some Commentary

There is a point where we can see therapeutic and educational strategies as interventionist, because they are not allowing the energy to find its own way. There appears to be a massive imposition of old stress and established tracking patterns which occurs from the very beginning of life when the initial infantile energy is chaotic or, even more intriguingly, is already determinedly and prenatally implanted.

So many educators in schools want success, easeful learning, easeful teaching, simple, mindless retraumatization, and indoctrination, not dwelling on impossible problems in learning. In a hopefully bottoming-out century of violence and despair, it seems the most important part of what schools can do is to face what constitutes learning and what lessons are worth learning. That these might be about invisibility and immobility would hardly suit most supervisory school committees.

When the energy does find its own way, we are amazed at its fluidity, its speed, its complexity, its genius. We must relocate ourselves within this free movement, yet not from our ordinary, narrative ways of approaching freedom or our experiences of freedom.

Rather, apparently, freedom can be regained from the most difficult place of recognition, from the place in the held-energy system at which we as some kind of space traveller, have landed. This usually occurs when we realize we are in some kind of deeper suffering that requires going beyond the usual methods we try to alleviate ordinary pain.

Our centering process, as it has been called, amounts to (re)discovering the core energetic and following its directions, almost; well, as best as we can. The obvious and not so obvious encumbrances to achieving this connection (covenant) are well documented by spiritual and religious strategies throughout the ages. As noted before, even specialized breathing techniques such as found in yoga modalities, which might seem rock bottom simple, or if not simple, at least primally basic, may be, at the energetic level I am talking about, an imposition, a retraumatization.

Frieda

The core of the problem for me is staying out of the way of the energy. We have to allow it to proceed along its assigned, self-unlocking path. While doing this energy work, when I ask her, "Tell me what you sense," Frieda, in her early fifties, always remarks, "Tell me what you want me to say."

Some time later, by way of contextualizing this remark, she complains that there is too much going on for her in her awareness during a session to discriminate what is important, what is relevant, and what is not. She then turns back to her process and tells me what she sees energetically, including scenes from former lives replete with castles and dungeons, and (soap-)operatic relationships.

Frieda faces the general problem of making the transition into the energetic. She does not think it relevant to the pains in her belly, or the chronic twitches in her legs. Her brain glances at the color forms and then her attention swoops down upon them, overwhelming the energy with narrative, interpretation, historical and imaginative elaborations. These "horizontal" observations do not accompany the vertical movement which signals change.

Levine might call these mental and verbal "phrases" titrations, momentary pausing places where the toxicity of the trauma is diluted before the traumatic pattern is confronted again. He appears to align with these elaborations and encourages them.

I have gotten confused about this, because I recall some practitioners saying that these are places of resistance to energetic movement, based upon fear. There is an implied judgment that the creative value espoused, namely of free-flowing energy, must be released; and anything short of that carries a burden of shame and guilt with it, for both client and practitioner.

If Frieda elaborates because she cannot tolerate energetic movement, she even may be wedded to the narrative produced in response to held-energy systems, because it is the only way to stop the flowing, or to dampen it. Significantly abused by her parents, as an anxious, racing neurochemistry, Frieda experiences the immobilizations as refuges, life-rafts for the definition of self, floating above a deeper, more turbulent chemical ocean. The long and short of it is that these horizontal elaborations keep Frieda distracted in a false prison from which she is (falsely) always trying to free herself. At the crux, colloquially noted, there is not enough space within for her to allow herself to be.

Frieda's observing brain offers fanciful, accurate, and insightful observations about former lives, and rooms, and situations of jealousy and the like. It has the quality of an imaginative genius elaboration on something only fragmentally observed, the momentary perception of energy in the abstract forms of color. Yet because at the center of the problem is black, and brain reads that as dangerous, she often does not follow whatever color there is directly to a black center.

Yet it seems that all resolving movement in held energy begins at black, within black. So I reply to Frieda, "Don't put me in that role of telling you what to say. Then you can set me up as the bad guy, whom you then can oppose. That's not what this procedure is about." If we can't sense the difference between titrations (detoxifying horizontal resting stations) and the vertical moves into the transforming matrix of the black, we can, as many therapists do, stay with our clients in those secondary levels of titration and insight and never evoke change or sense what it really looks like.

After many sessions of this I finally find the words. I tell Frieda, "OK, if you want me to tell you what to do, stay out of the way of the energy!" That stills her static-filled process, and she and I bemusedly watch her brain try to deal with my perhaps koan.

Held energy must be held. For most people, and for brain, the only change which appears significant is the change from black energy into color, from patterns which hold, into awareness which is clear. Brain appears not interested in any other kind of change, an interesting social thought, grounded in our experience of the repetitive, cyclical patterns of social change which do not change the fundamental "human" patterns of suffering, war, and peace.

Suffering

I intuit suffering reflects a traumatic conundrum, wherein our brain cannot find its way out of the traumatic pattern. Brain returns to the neurochemistry evoked by the held-energy system as a way of trying to find the point of traumatic origin (Levine's T_0), without knowing it is in traumatic process. Both Buddha and Christ consciousness (neurochemistry) strategize that there are ways out of the patterns of suffering, that suffering is not a permanent and required necessity. These strategies involve giving up self or ego, which, under these rubrics, are based upon narrative, variously identified as illusion, attachment, ignorance, sin, etc.

The experiences of feeling states, such as happiness, sadness, anger, may be interesting, but they do not take us directly into the deepest levels of energetic wherein change occurs. I remind clients they can witness their feelings, but not to spend a lot of time in them, or even emoting them, as we have been taught to do in therapies these days.

There are individuals who have felt that getting in touch with their feelings is the end-all of therapy. I ask my clients, "Did that ever help you to change?" The bemused response is, "No, not with the patterns which have remained in place." Feelings are a piece of the puzzle, and for those who have not learned about feelings, they may patterns which have remained in place." Feelings are a piece of the puzzle, and for those who have not learned about feelings, they may be crucial to taking responsibility. But rarely do I hear that that strategy has brought permanent change to the current patternings that preoccupy the clients I see.

As for guilt and shame, these states or chemistries may obscure the real nature of traumatic process and confound the completion usually characterized by a rubric involving forgiveness. Forgiveness and compassion may be experiences, but the point of origin for the traumatic patterns is energetic, not emotional. Years of emotional work may prepare for change, but emotion does not prompt it, at least for those clients whose patterns persist.

Language and Energy

I am in my own process after a week in Boulder, where I experience so much, it is hard to say what sticks and what does not. My work with clients, eager to join me in the search, are perhaps the greatest part of my own healing. A couple of points stand out among many.

One, the maintenance of language and narrative can be a way of perpetrating the status quo. Language is a resting place, before the ascent/descent into the non-verbal. It has a horizontal quality, a latitude which in fact limits, and proscribes. It does not describe, in the way that what is being described is describable. Or worth describing. The sense of moving into cellular memory is expansive and radiates to the end of the universe, whereas language takes us to tiny places (not unimportant).

A diamond placed upon my forehead sets off the tiniest of pains, a filigree thread of gossamer headache across the back of my brain. Its subtlety is remarkable as is my new-found capacity to intuit that on some level, this sequence may be most significant.

When we titrate held-energy systems' toxicity, we hover in the status quo, before going on. My psychoanalysis was not about change, but about consolidation, or preservation of the status quo, holding until I could go on. I wanted change, or said I did, but I was afraid. I hold my analysis to account for generating my own awareness of the difference between stasis and movement.

Taking Responsibility

I was talking with Roland, aged 15, about situations where there has been victimization, such as in cases of child abuse. We noted generally how we start as victims, then as victims, we somehow sometimes become perpetrators (he had). I added, "If I see perpetrators as victims, which I agree they are, I don't know what it means to take responsibility."

Roland offered, "To take responsibility means to see the pattern of victimization and perpetration, and to stop them both, externally as well as internally." Responsibility, we conjectured, means to see how the pattern has been taken up, over generations, and to hold it while it melts or self-dissolves, a sign the information has been integrated. What to do, even in the worst cases (they are always the worst)? The answer, not new, is a very special kind of witnessed nothing.

A Moment in the Day

Yesterday, the scan of an arrow halfway down the shaft starts to melt, and I am apprehensive about what that will do to me. Will it make the erection possible, or impossible? Yet I breathe free into the cells after staying with my anxiety for a time. My cells contain a dance of molecules and within those particles lies my freedom. I must experience energy's transforming essence.

If I breathe with awareness of every cell, I now wonder whether I can transform the metabolic holding pattern which creates my extra weight.

Media Reportage and Energy

When we hear of a president dropping his pants before a kneeling woman, both vulnerable to the narrative of power, we think we are finding something out, some secret we did not know. But this kind of "information" is already characterized, is itself a retraumatization and without delicate and probing focus, is retraumatizing. In the media such information occurs with regularity in recurring horizontal formulations along apparently safe vectors, with no plunge into the vertical, into the black.

The newspaper stories read the same, and still we have not found out directly how the black is approached, or in what contexts of trust (athletic, political, religious, artistic?) connection with it can be achieved. We never find out what is going on, what immobility the president and his hotel consort are experiencing. By exposing a dirty "truth," we are being confirmed in illusion.

If we are looking for a definition of progress, must we not attend at this level? Otherwise, we will be continually surprised when, in response to trust, like maybe being elected president, or securing power as dictator of a country, brain of leader offers up its trauma for resolution. I think the current revelations about public figures require more, delicate focus in the area of what is being learned and what is traumatically fixed, not less.

Political and religious leaders carry and perpetrate their held-energy patterns as the rest of us do, which is all the time until we experience moments of our self-liberating neurochemistry. Thus we need to know what patterns these leaders are working on, so that as in a marriage, we can identify which phase of their healing we are participating in. Hobbes argues for the expression of government as commonwealth in the figure of a single personality. This is one way to identify how as body politic, we have joined with them in community wherein we agree that they are the leaders.

Why should we as the public get drawn into situations where the (potentially self-destructive) pattern is perpetrated in its most impossible immobility by individuals who, in the full flush of trust, are least inclined to penetrate the black they have unwittingly brought forward? I suspect for many, their understanding of power, granted through election or otherwise, implies the permission to bring the patterns forward, even to project and transfer them to the common weal.

The secret ambition their eros propels them toward could be energetic completion within political narrative, and we give them permission. And will we continue ending up outside some bunker, raking through ashes for signs of some lesson learned, when nothing has been learned?

Technique Hallmarks

The following are hallmarks of this **held-energy systems** (trauma completion) technique:

1. The effects of trauma can be expressed at many levels—psychic, psychological, personality, physical, and spiritual, for examples. Until recently, trauma patterning was perceived to be centered in active, blocked memory, or to perpetuate from some invisible realm (the unconscious), or from the body. However, it also can reside at some subtle energy level, in those cases where it cannot be otherwise completed nor can behavior, insight, or thought patterns change it. Trauma patterning can reside in the forms of **held-energy systems,** which we have not been able to look at directly, because we did not know where or how to look.

2. To gain access to the energetic realms and their landscapes, brain must proceed to a vibrational level—here, with this technique, by focusing upon color and shapes, which are then examined closely and witnessed. Other vibrational, sensate capabilities can also be used.

3. With energetic support from an appropriate and non-intentional surround (practitioner's holding touch), brain immediately offers up its traumatic patterning (in **held-energy systems**). Some patterns are

harder to accommodate to neurochemically; they appear toxic and need to be addressed in slow fashion.

4. This technique/perspective teaches how to find and focus upon **held-energy systems**, characterized by black, and "bruised" energy, characterized by brown. We do not spend a lot of time in narrative—story, memory, emotional release—these more traditional focusing modes approximate, even represent and express the **held-energy systems**, but more often do not allow for completion or dissolution of the pattern of the system.

5. We assume brain can focus upon any level of magnification in the mindbody to resolve a **held-energy system** and by intrapolation, a neurochemistry. The practitioner can guide the focus of the client to any level which they both sense is appropriate.

6. This technique/perspective teaches how to *follow the directions on the package*, to take the material in the order brain seems to want to study the pattern. If we are to get to a prime, spindle trauma, we must allow brain to tell the story in its order, not ours. To this effect, no intention or will should be conveyed. Client and practitioner get out of the way and merely focus and watch what happens.

At the end of the session, there can be the sense that something significant has occurred, but that neither client nor practitioner has "done anything." **Any** superimposition of breathing, special posture, or interpretation template, theory, or technique is evaluated for retraumatization. Locating this initiating intuition is critical for completing our most fundamental trauma patterns.

7. This technique/perspective does not use hypnosis or trance modes. Both client and practitioner can move comfortably with commentary, observation, laughter, then return to the energetic. "Suggestion," by default and inexperience, may occur, but both client and therapist come to see the error this involves. They can watch out for that and

return to the more difficult position being attended to which interpretation or suggestion, as interventions, offer as substitute.

8. This technique/perspective shows how the brain can generalize and extrapolate to widespread, systemic completions from the specific and vice versa. If brain solves one particulate form, then many are solved.

9. The purposes of this technique/perspective are to experience how trauma is stored and completed in the mindbody. The basic mechanisms include: the held-energy systems contained in black; the protective and confounding pushing-away phenomenon in the area surrounding black; the transformation of neurochemistry, witnessed; the way in which focusing at the energetic level places us at the source or access point of the patterns which most people describe as physiological symptoms, the interface of subtle energy and body.

At the point of incarnation, where the energetic appears dense and solid, this translation becomes "visible," and brain can see how narrative keeps us in the pattern. The movement of the mind/brain into the energetic allows brain to solve its most difficult problems with everybody standing back to watch it, but within a matrix of full, boundaried, non-intentional, proximal, and surrounding energetic support.

10. This technique/perspective apparently can be done lying down and with physical contact at the neck or at other places on the body. Physical movement by the client may distort client focus where the pattern has a particular physical torque, so remaining still is often the best way to bring the *meditational*, energetic aspect of this work to the fore.

With adolescents in a school setting and where boundaries are of particular concern, it can be attempted using pencil and paper across a table.

11. Risks:

1. Possible disorientation from reconfiguring of neurochemistry, including experiences approximating mild intoxication, changes in blood pressure, reactivation of trauma compression, emergence of deeper, more difficult patterning as a result of reconfiguring and dissolving more superficial ones.

2. Some surprising and immediate physical and psychological changes, such as dropped addictions, removed chronic thought patterns, resolution of physical, developmental, and psychodynamic relational hiatus. These experiences can lead to

3. Increased sense of personal, spiritual efficacy which may lead to a sense that the world of people is more out of control, more substantially dissociated than is safe.

4. Getting clear rather more easily than we thought possible makes us wonder about our substructures of personality and their spiritual limits.

CHAPTER SIX: A SESSION

An initial session begins with a discussion of trauma theory. I am not particularly interested initially in developing anything as grandiose as narrative understanding. I do ask about traumata, including sexual abuse or abuse of any kind, confirming that there will be none in this setting. I tell anecdotes about the risks and responses of clients to the work.

In a return session, a client may tell me about what has happened in the explorations of this different way of experiencing. Someone needing additional therapeutic support is usually involved in some other modality, or can be referred. For these purposes, I do not contract as primary therapist, a role I believe to be traditionally full of intention. My function is meditational and educational, instructing brain how to witness and solve its own process.

For those clients who have been Rolfed, or who are in a Rolfing series, we experiment with alternating sections of Rolfing touch and intention with the energy work. Rolfing can help to ground the client. It provides the opportunity to witness the incarnation of the energy at sensate levels. Most initial Rolfees remain with the Rolfing recipe until the first series is concluded.

At the beginning of a session, the client lies face up, the top of the head abutting the edge of one end of the table. I place the lower legs on a cushion, to provide support and eliminate fatigue. I usually cover the body to hold heat because we are encouraging minimal movement. I explain, "If you can move without changing the energy patterns you are scanning, OK, then move. But if your movement is a commentary on, rebellion against, or completion of the energy problem you are witnessing, then don't. Let your brain solve this problem energetically without movement."

Synopsis

In this session, the client, a woman bodyworker in her mid-twenties whom I shall call Grace, examines a trauma pattern which includes, according to her narrative, a near-drowning incident when she was a very young child. The incident does not become recognizable to her or to me until well into the session. Prior to that, we hover in patterning, trying to establish the architecture of where we are, and sensing how to proceed (within minute 5, at line 54: hereafter noted 5/54). By minute 7, line 88 (7/88), we have begun to see the beginnings of the main episodion which she describes. She focuses for a while upon a green vibration until 10/155, when the configuration shifts.

At 12/180 she goes deeper toward some core. We are able to deal with the black and the structures it appears in and what it contains. By line 14/214, she has entered it completely. By 16/262, the image of drowning occurs. The near-death experience appears at 18/284. A significant part of the completion of the energetic action occurs by 22/362.

By 24/394, the narrative form of the drowning begins to emerge. By 25/414, a recognition occurs, with various aftermath insights and connections, including 29/468. With a new alignment toward some completion, Grace heads "down a vortex." I believe this movement approximates the serious action that dissociative process, including tragic forms, seeks to describe.

She continues into the held-energy system, evoking narrative which includes an historical memory of near-drowning. Through 39/645, she meditates in the extremity of the chemistry conundrum. By 44/726, significant change is occurring, as one of the bubble forms turns into a cedar box. By 46/750, the form produces a medicine healing "companion" spirit in the form of a bear.

Grace hovers in the narrative of her relationship to the bear, then we head back into the vibrational energetic at 49/791. By 53/840, Grace experiences a stress pattern relief, as a landscape greens, and the neurochemistry balances. Line 54/856 initiates an interpretive, analytic reworking of the data and the evaluation of what she has accomplished. By 59/931, we begin to separate in a series of non-retraumatizing exchanges. Various commentaries and post-game chalktalk fill the conclusion of the session.

Please note: Because of printing convention, the table-like form I have used necessitates that you now turn the book on its side.

At the left of each page, each change in dialogue voice is numbered, and in the first cell of the table on the left, the voices are identified: **Client** is identified by **C**, and **Practitioner** by **P**. In the next column to the left is the dialogue itself. I have placed asterisks [*] in the dialogue text at approximately fifteen-second intervals, because I think it might be interesting to note how long some of these transformations take.

I have set the narrow middle column to indicate the total time sequence in minutes and fifteen second intervals. The placements are roughly accurate and are there to give an overall sense where in the progress of the session things happen.

I have also indicated where the tape is inaudible or where there are possible variations in the transcription with brackets ([-]) and markings [???]. This session, conducted over two years ago, is representative for illustrative purposes, and I am planning publishing more controlled sessions in the future, which will include refinements of technique, or better, absence of technique, as well as more complete transcription.

In the far righthand column, I comment on the dialogue, sometimes referring by number to the lines which illustrate the sequence I am describing. Where there are particular highlights on basic premises of this technique, I have placed [**]. My suggestion is to listen to the tape [where applicable] with the text on the left, then read the commentary at the right side of the page.

Please note that because of space and desktop publishing computer programming considerations, only odd-number pages are numbered, and the lower margins of the table vary according to the marginal wisdom of the word-processing program.

I am particularly grateful to the wonderful spirit and playful intelligence of my client, a colleague.

			0:00																

1	C:	That should be on the (front).	0:00
2	P:	Um-hum [OK.].	
3	C:	And darkness here on this.	
4	P:	Um-hum [OK.].	
5	C:	And gray.	
6	P:	Um-hum [OK.]. Is there spatially a relationship between those elements?*	0:15
7	C:	Uh-huh [Yes.]. Let me show you. [Gesture]. We have a bubble coming out of darkness. And it's just really gray.	
8	P:	Uh-huh [OK.]. OK, that's got a curve to it.	
9	C:	Uh-huh [Yes.].	
10	P:	All right. And then it's, it's surrounded by gray.* Is it, is it surrounded on all sides by gray?	0:30
11	C:	Not underneath.	

TRAUMA ENERGETICS

169

12	P:	Not underneath.		
13	C:	It's like a drip or something.		
14	P:	A drip. OK. So what's		
15	C:	And as we're talking, it's receding.		
16	P:	Yeah. [Laugh].* It's not going to stick around.	0:45	
17	C:	No, not really, no.		
18	P:	Uh-huh [OK.]. Is it replaced by anything or is it just		
19	C:	I don't know. It's just, it gets replaced by more white and gray.* It's like every time I talk it moves up and then down.	1:00	Somehow there is a connection between speech and the form or pattern which is being addressed.
20	P:	Yes.		
21	C:	Um.		
22	P:	Let's try an experiment here. Why don't, why don't you, uh,* if, if by not talking and not moving into the speech centers of the brain, you can just hold the image, I'll try to guide you	1:15	Intuitively, I suggest that she talk as little as necessary. The strategy that she can choose to stay out of speech centers in order to focus elsewhere, is just introduced. The process is shared, between practitioner and client. My objective is to demystify this work, and to stay intuitively in touch with client's "process."
23	C:	Umum. [OK.].		

24	P:	And if it's gray, just lift your finger, to acknowledge that* it's followable. OK? Now, let's follow the point.	1:30	Finger signals keep the communication to kinesthetic level. Not all clients do it quite this way—this way emerged here, and I have used it rarely since.
25	C:	Uh-huh.		
26	P:	I don't know if this will work, but it's, we'll, uh.... So you've got some gray, in front of you. Good.* Why don't you lift your finger now just to say yes or to try it [indicate]. And I want you to [???]think of it. See if you can enter the gray. Stay out of speech.* There. And see if you now can go, see if you can go deeper into the, is the gray like a cloud or a vapor?	1:45 2:00	26-30. In trauma, the ordinary relationship between speech and energetic experience seems to be compromised. While speech is used a lot, it is not the primary mode of experiencing. **Gray is a key color. Whenever it is located, usually it can be entered as a color, a "zoom shot" into the canvas of a painting, as it were, where at a micro level, it can be divided into particles of black and white, the former then viewed and discussed as to what needs to happen. Brain seems to be able to move up and down the ladder of magnification, to divide the problem into component "digestible" parts.
27	C:	[Gestures "Yes."]		

TRAUMA ENERGETICS

28	P:	So let's go toward....* If you can do a pointillist, you know the way the Seurat's paintings, you know, makes [paints] all the dots that then make up the colors. Or like a newspaper, if you take a magnifying glass and go in, you know,* to one of the pictures. And if you look close, it's made up of white and black, making up the gray, right? So what I want you to do is to go into the gray at a,[???] at a microscopic level and find *a dot, of black. All right. See what you can find that.	2:15 2:30 2:45	** Often client will feel a pushing away energy, characterized emotionally as a reluctance or a fear, to confront the black. We remain at the vectorial level rather than the emotional. I explain that I see this pushing away as the neurochemical warning signal to stay away from this nexus of held energy. Reportedly, brain reads this signal ten times a second, yet because it is coded in black, it cannot enter. Like a Kafka situation, brain is troubled by this traffic bump, yet when it looks at it directly, it is as if the door is locked, or repeating the approach, the wall is sealed over. The more directly we approach traumatically held-energy systems at the verbal, meaning, or emotional levels, the more confounded brain process appears to become. The various aspects or qualities of black noted by brain (shiny, matte, hard, rough, porous, etc.) all have a punlike quality or set of associations, but rarely do I move into the speech or analytic modes of functioning during the session, even to "enjoy" a Freudian joke with the client. When I do, it seems a mistake, and clients will remind me that it is when I do it; they report such commentary takes them out of their focusing. We stay in the concreteness of the language as an avenue to abandoning language and focusing relatively unencumbered upon the held energy by entering or sampling the color.
29	C:	[Gestures "Yes."]		
30	P:	And it's in view?*	3:00	
31	C:	[Gestures "Yes."]		

32	P:	And you get, can you go in close to it? Or is it sort of, [Gesture???]there, you're close to it?* And is it, is it round, or is it just round, or is it angled?	3:15	I am trying to explore my understanding about the nature of "brain's" delineation of the problem: What is the size, density, and shape of the conjoining vectors as imaged? Here the image always is considered a secondary presentation of deeper forces in the chemistry.
33	C:	Round.		"Round" offers a number of directions to go in—to the circumferential edge, to the center, to the underside, to the relationship of front (top) to back (bottom), to something circumscribed, to some image of wholeness, or even to rationality. Here I ask polite questions as a part of my interest in the energetic experience. Whatever the approach we take, we stay away from meaning, symbol, verbal-insight understanding.
34	P:	It's round. Good. So now at this point we can maybe try going in and speak to that.* Is that all right? Is it, it doesn't, we're not just going[???]in?	3:30	
35	C:	No.		
36	P:	OK, so that, we're OK. So let's go to the.... Tell me something about its structure[???] Is it hard? Is it dense, or is it....*	3:45	I start to give focusing leadership, then pull back. I want to find out what brain is offering up. In held-energy systems, the brain chemistry seems to consolidate and objectify the energy. The description of its nature by the brain tells us something about its difficulty, neurochemically speaking (this is hard, this is dense, this has a cutting edge, etc.).

37	C:	I think it's pretty heavy.[???] [Gestures size.]		
38	P:	It's like a ping pong. Can you magnify the, the ping pong and take a closer look at it and see what,* what is possible there.[???]	4:00	** As noted before, I believe the brain scans to varying levels of magnification in our mindbody, and it monitors these constantly. The client utilizes this magnification capacity and accepts it as true. Our ordinary "awareness" aligns whatever awareness is with that innate capacity, hence the power of directed magnification as a technique. Various brain strategies which are otherwise inexplicable become visible as one spelunks through the chemistry.
39	C:	It's hard for me to do that[???inaudible] for some reason.		
40	P:	Yes.		
41	C:	And what I'm feeling is that there's this blackish[???]* stuff moving in[???] over here.	4:15	**Mind or consciousness is not doing the work. In fact, all ego in the intentional sense is being challenged here to stay out of the way of brain process. Our power here is in observation. The free association of Freud, depending upon the primacy of the insight, symbolic, and verbal meaning-related processes, is here excluded from the main course of the experiential meal. For those patterns which have not been resolved by language, and emotive therapies, something more disciplined and perhaps simply austere may be required. Brain must confront what is difficult in its purest form, as it initially confronted the trauma which sets in the held-energy chemistry which it now finds so problematic.
42	P:	Right.		

43	C:	But I'm (um[???]).... So I can pull that point in, but I can't, um, keep it there.		When the pattern of black wanders or cannot be "speared" or fixed, like an unruly hors d'oeuvre, the force of the neurochemical prohibition surrounding black is experienced not as resistance, which may be its emotional, intellectual counterpart, but as a phenomenon; the client then senses the movement toward as well as away from the black, and other points of focus or approaches have to be considered. Many of these are typical and familiar to the client.
44	P:	You can't keep it there. Good. So that's a straight kind* of a [process???]. That's, that's what it looks like, you know, the brain says, "It's too dangerous," or , "It's too difficult, or	4:30	I find myself repeating what the client has said to make sure that I have the problem right, as the client has presented it. I guess I confirm the neurochemical position and validate its importance, then offer a strategy.
45	C:	Uhn-huuh [OK.].		
46	P:	"I don't know how to handle this, so I better stay out of it. It's going to screw up the rest of the chemistry there."		
47	C:	Well, I can't.		Client acknowledges the place chemistry won't allow "her" to go.

#	Speaker	Utterance	Time	Commentary
48	P:	So that's, * you're looking straight at [traumatic] for now. This is, in, in analytic terms people would say, "Well, that's resistance," you know,	4:45	48-52. With clients who are professional mental health or helper-type people, I feel I show off a bit, but also the effort is to ease both of us out of analytic modes into pure energetics. Often they will substitute comments like this one. Her response indicates that my comment may be premature, or irrelevant. I am trying to teach my strategy (we can move from analytic modes to energetic) before it presents itself. Maybe my comment sets a platform, maybe not.
49	C:	Uh-huh [tentative OK.].		
50	P:	But I don't think that's useful.		I head toward indicating how the mode of focus and registering what is experienced is physical.
51	C:	Un-huh [tentative OK.].		
52	P:	It's, it's just, you know, it's just physical [difficult???].		I give words to confirm the level from which I think it best to focus. For clients stuck in words, which often happens in traumatic patterning, this approach may reduce the process to its essence.
53	C:	Uh-huh [OK.].		
54	P:	Can you, * can you go, can you go behind the pinpoint?	5:00	54-58. Once the point of engagement in the pattern begins to consolidate, the architecture of the situation clarifies, and we discover natural questions emerging. If the brain balks, we knows that our approach "etiquette" needs to be refocused.
55	C:	All around.		

56	P:	You can go all around it; good. All around it. Does it look any different from the back than from the front?	
57	C:	Um-um [No.].	
58	P:	The same.	
59	C:	It's, it's flat, though, *like a, thicker than a button, but, but, um, it's not like a button.	5:15	**Held-energy systems can appear in many forms, some more solid than others. I intuit that all forms essentially resolve in a dissolution or completion from within. Any superimposition of motive, intention, will, or visualization which does not stay with the problem brain is really having with the pattern may be retraumatizing or maintaining the status quo. Any offer of interpretation of meaning is counterproductive to renegotiating (Levine's term) the pattern. When the client is analytically trained and is used to processing information that way, then the task is to offer him/her this additional mode of energetic experiencing. As clients get the feel of the importance of this approach, and gain confidence in "going for the black," they seek out the difficulty, rather than avoid it. Here the system is flat, with some thickness or depth, perhaps a connecting piece. The brain will pun or in other ways give clues—but again, it is not this strategy to hover at a meaning or narrative, or symbolic level. (Continued next cell).

60	P:	It's thicker than a button but not not like a button.		*(Continued from above cell).* The client moves through the clarified version of the "object" (objectified energy). I think brain reads the energy and within the "last" instant, attaches a coded label in some recognizable form. My strategy is to "deconstruct" that and stay at the energetic, including its difficulties and impasses.
61	C:	It's kind of....There's* more of it around the circumference.	5:30	
62	P:	Yep [Yes.]. Yeah [OK.]. Can you zoom in any closer?		I use the strategy of zooming in and out like a microscope or a zoom lens on a camera, or like some space traveller heading in and out of some planetary entity.
63	C:	Like a space ship.		
64	P:	Yes, it's [just???] like a space ship, and is it, and it...Can you move in any closer to it?*	5:45	
65	C:	Uh-huh [Yes.].		
66	P:	Good. How are the, are, when you say space ship, does it have lights in it or is it		I am not certain whether we are talking about my idea of taking a space ship like a space traveller approaching a space station, or whether the button is the space ship. I try to clarify. Sometimes my own stuff gets in the way. When I have done this with adolescent students face to face across a desk (where I am not touching and they draw the images they sense), this kind of confusion does not happen.
67	C:	Um-um [No.].		
68	P:	No. So it's, it's just a shape		

69	C:	Uh-huh [Yes.].	
70	P:	that you're looking at. Could you go to the surface of it and tell me what you see?	
71	C:	*It's like a that, that [gesture], unh, hidden whatever the [???surface] has a resiliency or whatever's, like a car.	6:00
72	P:	It's like a car. It's a hard surface.	
73	C:	Uh-huh [Yes.].	
74	P:	Is it, can you* intuit whether the center is also hard? Is it all the way that like a.... Or is it, is it like a car that has a, you know....	6:15
75	C:	There's space inside.	With focus, brain can penetrate held-energy systems, even though at times it thinks it cannot, because on some level it accepts what it sees at "face value."
76	P:	There's space inside. Good.	I confirm the knowledge because it sounds accurate, and it comes immediately in response to my question. There is no kind of prevarication, as far as I can tell. It also presents a more complex reality than was initially known. I would say brain here is beginning to resolve the black in part by penetrating it with no intention to destroy it, but to focus merely.

TRAUMA ENERGETICS

179

A SESSION

#				
77	C:	But the* shell's real thick.	6:30	Once a shell appears, we have the architecture of inner and outer, and there are focusing maneuvers which can be invoked to clarify the interface between inner and outer, all of which may have resonances to cellular as well as to gross body structure or even psychological boundaries. None of these levels is approached as such.
78	P:	The shell's real thick.		
79	C:	And the space just feels, just a small part of it on the inside.		
80	P:	Right. Can you intuit if there's a color in the space or there's anything you sense, an acknowledge —		I move, perhaps too abruptly for my own sense of order, to the vibrational level. Months after this session, I now set up that strategy as an expectation or formula. I say, "Let's see if we can move to the vibrational level—can you scan for light or darker densities or is there color in the situation you are viewing?"
81	C:	Well,		
82	P:	an acknowledge[ment]....		
83	C:	when you said that I got a* light green.	6:45	
84	P:	A light green.		
85	C:	But it, there was only that flash through it. It was still, almost like it was clear in there, but then it got that flash of light green.		
86	P:	Yeah [OK.].		

87	C:	flash of light green.		
88	P:	So this is, this is, this is a structure. This is an energetic place, you know,* of some interest.	7:00	88-92. I offer a strategy for focusing, without standard "interpretation." There are varieties of green, and my first sense is that it is a diluted color, perhaps the green is a "green light," or an acknowledgement of movement, or because of the flash, a toxic pattern, or some kind of neurological spiking.
89	C:	Uhmhm [Yes.].		
90	P:	Something is, is inside[???] there is, brain is trying to characterize it there as being contained[???with the green].		
91	C:	Uh-huh [Yes.].		
92	P:	Is it, can you go towards the* surface of the black, the car-like....	7:15	I return to the manifest problem in the form brain offers it. Let's see if there are further details. Every focusing is made toward greater clarification of what is, but under the neurochemical rubric of black, the focus is directed toward a neurochemically forbidden territory. Each new assimilation of information suggests a transformation of the neurochemistry of trauma, which involves the energetic vectors of approach and avoidance, often documented in other ways by psychology, at the message of black.
93	C:	And magnify it?		
94	P:	Yeah, magnify it or....		

#	Speaker	Utterance	Time	Commentary
95	C:	Uh-huh [Yes.].		
96	P:	What does it look like at the surface?*	7:30	
97	C:	Um, real porous, uh, light* travelling through it	7:45	97-107. It seems brain works on the problem of understanding the information originally perceived as a button shape. Light begins to enter and transform the system.
98	P:	Umum [OK].		
99	C:	uh, all the way out.		
100	P:	Umum [OK].		
101	C:	Still very hard.		
102	P:	But there is light traveling through it?*	8:00	
103	C:	There are little tiny pinpoints.		
104	P:	Yeah [OK]. Had you seen that before?		
105	C:	No.		
106	P:	So this is new information?		**I offer a strategy for understanding the change which brain is manifesting. Structures approached in this way can become instruments of information which can then be absorbed and renegotiated and absorbed. Again, this is a formula of focus, namely of learning what is here. This is what makes this approach educational, not therapeutic.
107	C:	Uh-huh [Yes.].		

108	P:	OK. So let's go toward, uh what should we do? Should we go through toward the, uh,*	8:15	
109	C:	Middle?		
110	P:	middle? Let's try to understand that and see if we can give brain a chance to figure what that's about.		I am maintaining the ascetic style here, so that intentionality and traditional "ego" functioning does not take over and absorb the information, thereby distracting brain from heading for the most troubling held-energy systems.
111	C:	There's something contained in there whose???, um,* if you go through one of th' little pipes inside....	8:30	111-132. Continuing brain process as the pattern becomes more prominent, including within it, problematic areas which cannot be easily resolved. The appearance of red suggests healing, anger, heat, passion, intensity, and the like. The bubble suggests a thinness of boundary, perhaps thinness of "defense," but something which can be seen through. The initial opacity of the surface ("hard") is now perceived as thin and perhaps fragile, pop-able.
112	P:	Yeah [OK].		
113	C:	It, I never saw something on the inside. But on the inside, it's, it's, um,* it's like a bubble; there's, there's people or something insi[de], or humans inside.	8:45	Brain is clarifying the objectified, held energy into something more fragile, less severe, more integrated, more human.
114	P:	Yeah [OK].		
115	C	Um, there's something red.* Somebody's wearing red.	9:00	

116	P:	Um-hum [OK.].		
117	C:	And there's entities or things in [and???], um, a people mingling.		
118	P:	Umum [OK.].		
119	C:	Um.* The surface is flattening so that I can get closer just where I am.	9:15	The ridge is flattening out—the declension of the trauma is hard to read here, whether we are seeing something resolve or we are going to the center immobility (Levine's *To*). Riding this wave flexibly seems to be the best way: letting the brain offer its examination in its own order.
120	P:	Um-hum [OK.].		
121	C:	And then kind of coming back around a little.		
122	P:	Yep [Yes.].		
123	C:	Um.		
124	P:	*So something in the cha[nge], the, the brain is understanding this in a different way, isn't it?	9:30	
125	C:	Uh-huh [Yes.]. It's not letting me move in.		
126	P:	Yeah [Yes.].		
127	C:	And the black comes back around it.		
128	P:	Umum [OK.].		

129	C:	But I, I haven't yet gotten in to the circle, or into* the, the bubble.	
130	P:	Right.	9:45
131	C:	Um, I'm right up against the bubble.	
132	P:	Is this almost like a, an M&M? You're in still,	

** I try to find an easily accessible image to confirm what I am hearing so that I can orient myself. Sometimes a client will feel how my suggestion determines too much what her/his brain subsequently offers on the screen. It is as if I am suggesting, and brain wants to please, so offers back what I have asked for. But the dialogue and the trust involved seems to support even my "mistakes," which, if misleading, are quickly reworked by brain. I proffer the strategy as strategy, delivering it in a bit of a rush to keep my connection for experiencing the structure being witnessed by the client. We both agree to use the example of "M&M" (my example, but taken from her hand gestures and commentary) tentatively, to catalogue the energetic vectors, not the content of the image (sweet, chocolate, candy, etc.). What we are describing as an M&M is inaccurate, as it turns out—the bubble is not like an M&M, yet because the focus is upon surface and interior, approached from the interior, it seems an OK shorthand. We soon switch out of that. This is a common occurrence where I get it wrong. And invariably, the authority returns to the client, and ultimately to the energy. All the rest is strategy.

133	C:	Yes.	
134	P:	You're still in the,	
135	C:	Yeah [Yes.].	
136	P:	in th, what is it, the	
137	C:	The chocolate.	
138	P:	*You're heading toward the....	10:00
139	C:	Uh-huh [Yes.]. Uh-huh [Yes.].	
140	P:	Are we in the shell,	
141	C:	And you can....	
142	P:	or are we in the, are we in the...?	
143	C:	We're in the chocolate.	
144	P:	Uh-huh [OK.].	

#		Time	
145	**C:** And then the light green came back. And the light green now is, * is like the the, there's this funny light green color on the surface.	10:15	145-155. The relationship between inside and outside seems reworking here at some level. I support the movement—perhaps some clarification, so that the information contained in or of the green light is now appropriately on the outside, not the inside, where it had to be absorbed in this portion of the neurochemical system. The client may have taken in some pattern before she knew how to exclude it. The green light is toxic—or traumatically impacted, perhaps lightening up from black, or transitional, on its way to a deeper, more solid green.
146	**P:** On the surface now. It[We've???] reversed the, the...?		
147	**C:** Yeah, it just rev[ersed], the, the color.	10:30	
148	**P:** That's fantastic. I don't know what that means, but it sounds good.* (Laughter.)		
149	**C:** Yeah [Yes.].		
150	**P:** (Laughter.)		
151	**C:** A funny light green. Um....		
152	**P:** What is the, is the, now, here's a question. Uh, don't.... Tell me something about the funny light green. Say some more about it. Scan again. See if you can get another view of it,		
153	**C:** Well, it's		

TRAUMA ENERGETICS

A SESSION

154	P:		about it.
155	C:	10:45	*"it"'s, it's peelable. **When a surface peels, it peels by itself. When the client says, "I am peeling what is now peelable," I ask the client to return to focus on the peelability, but not on it being peeled. This is a major difference of approach to visualization therapists, such as psychosynthesists, who structure journeys through mountains, seeing wisemen, coming down the mountain—all of which in my experience have had a hasty, guided quality which do not allow the savoring of each part of the story. I have always fallen behind the guide, which in these critical places, left me "out of breath" and unable to focus on my own responses to the new material. Such guided journeys are interesting, and I have learned from taking them, but for me, they can be retraumatizations. They seem abusive to me in that they do not respect the order of the client brain in trauma. I suppose the broader message here is that brain, even when escorted to the proper viewing position, will not be able to negotiate the held-energy system on its own. It is my counter understanding that ultimately brain must be let alone in some critical way to recompute the information compressed in patterns located in held-energy systems.
156	P:		Yuh [Yes.].
157	C:		It now, I mean there's, it's like you can peel it. 157-163. Brain directs our process here. I am ready to move it along, but the client reports we have to stay where we are. I follow her(its) directive.
158	P:		It's peeling off. Or it can. It's peeling off.

159	C:	It can.		
160	P:	It can. It ha[s]....		
161	C:	It's still staying there, but it....		
162	P:	Why don't you just stay with it. Just look at the,* at the green color.		
163	C:	Um. That brings me out to where I'm floating above the green.	11:00	Focusing at a pure vibrational level brings a quick transformation: that the client can do this with no difficulty or hesitation suggests we are following the brain's story here, not ours, even though my M&M image, drawn from the original spaceship, does not exactly fit with the bubble. As practitioner with months more experience, I now might hover there with my own difficulty in blending the images, asking the client to check out her own sequence which engenders my confusion. If I am confused, the confusion may be shared.
164	P:	OK.		

#		Dialogue	Time	Commentary
165	C:	As I'm floating above the huge M&M in a way. And there's,		**The scale shifts in relationship to point of observation. An Alice in Wonderland "Drink me" phenomenon shows shifts in size and scale, some, I think, traumatically determined, some developmental. Proportionality of objects will suggest clues as to where in the developmental sequence or in the held-energy system we are. Here the object is huge, suggesting it is important, but not proportionate to the information it contains. The longer the brain stays in the difficulty of the problem and through time processes the pattern, the smaller it gets. Within this declining of scale, small may denote the information is more manageable.
166	P:	Right.		
167	C:	and there's, but there's space in the middle.		
168	P:	Right.		
169	C:	And um,* the green has variety.	11:15	The green (shell, if it is that) is no longer as rigidly constructed— the brain experiences its variety, which I underline. There may be a value vector I am expressing here. I don't do this quite as much now.
170	P:	Yes.		
171	C:	Um, like an M&M almost.		
172	P:	Uhn-huh [OK].		
173	C:	*Um, let's see.	11:30	

174	P:	That sounds, that's pretty good.		
175	C:	The green, a, but, um[???].* Um, the green's a holding.* The green's	11:45 12:00	The surrounding of a positive value vibration such as purple, white, even red, and here green, often appears to contain the deeper held-energy system in a partially protective sort of way, so that when brain scans the black, it reads: "Because the black is surrounded, it is in process, or its confounding nature, its spreading influence, is circumscribed. It is not bad black, it's OK—there's green there." In these situations, I have found that often a sharp delineation appears between the exterior surrounding color and the more problematic black interior. In a sense, the exterior green seems to be holding the inner stuff "in."
176	P:	Yeah [Yes,],		
177	C:	a*	12:15	
178	P:	yeah, isn't that interesting [what your seeing[???]?		
179	C:	a		
180	P:	I get that too. It's, it's protecting.		
181	C:	Yeah [Yes.].		
182	P:	Yeah, it's like,		
183	C:	Containing.		

#			Time	
184	P:	Yeah, it's containing this darker stuff, that's all. The dark stuff is, is, is that, is, is there a color to the dark stuff now? Is it black? There's a black with*	12:30	I ask the question. Currently I might wait for the black to be seen and so named without such prompting. As a practitioner, I sometimes sense a few steps ahead of the client. How this happens I don't know, except I often anticipate the sequence seconds, if not minutes ahead. Some of it is because the patterns become recognizable— people have similar energetic patterning. I also think it happens because of my physical, energetic contact with the client, and the fact that I am not necessarily similarly traumatized, so am not in the same dissociative patterns, though in the process, I intuit my energy field edges up to them like a tugboat to a steamer. But the boundary, confirmed by our physical contact, provides support, but not a push like a tugboat, nor a boundary cross-over into the client's system, so I think it is possible for me to read the information intuitively at a subtle energy level. Or in some subtle energetic combination beyond awareness, we co-influence and "agree" not to bring standard ego to our interface.
185	C:	It's been real black.		
186	P:	It's been real black,		
187	C:	Ick.		
188	P:	Yeah [Yes.].		
189	C:	It also has these elements of people with red dresses and things like that.		I begin to anticipate a literal scene here, perhaps a narrative of some incident, but brain will not move in so quickly.
190	C:	Uh-huh [OK.]. Uh-huh [OK.].		

191	P:	So that's part of it, but at a different level.		
192	C:	Uh-huh [OK.]. *And the black will do that, will flash on that deep purple, uh,* almost like it, it flashed on the deep purple and then it, and like the deep purple ran.	12:45 13:00	More healing vibrations get mixed up with other fragments, including red.
193	P:	Wow. Nice. Well, deep purple can be sort of a, I don't know, there are lots of interesting associations on that. It's not a bad color.		I give support in my own stunned way as I am impressed by the energies which are released by the approach into the black. I start but hesitate to give a meaning to the purple—not something I feel certain of in this context nor with my objective, which is to remain with the brain process on its own terms.
194	C:	Yeah [OK.].	13:15	
195	P:	*It's[???] got some healing in.		
196	C:	Uh-huh [Yes.].		
197	P:	It's vibrational stuff. But in the wrong order, it can, you can think you've got more than you've got.		197-199. Purple might imply some very high level (seventh chakra) wisdomy resolution which here seems jumping the gun—I sense brain is producing previews of coming conclusions, partially there, but not in sequence. With the client, I proffer a return to the green.
198	C:	Right.		
199	P:	Yeah [OK.]. So how's the green doing? How is....		

#		Utterance	Time	Notes
200	C:	It's just like a shellac.*	13:30	The green has a hard, perhaps translucent quality—it can be seen through to a deeper level—its protective (defensive?) quality is now of less interest to brain, which sees it as glossy (publicity shot?). Gloss suggests not just superficial sheen, but it often appears to reflect the beginning of movement, though the energy is still hardened.
201	P:	Yeah [Yes.]. Yeah [OK.].		
202	C:	That, umm,		
203	P:	It's just a, it's a gloss. It's a		
204	C:	Yeah [Yes.].		
205	P:	surface.		
206	C:	Yeah [Yes.].	13:45	
207	P:	Right. And are you, can you get close, closer* to it, or are you now still now at a distance?		
208	C:	It will let me go through it.		Here the brain finally masters the information and passes through it, in an order that seem sequential. At this point the surface becomes thin.
209	P:	Yes.		
210	C:	It will let me kind of move in and out of it, but it's just paper thin.		

211	P:	There we go. That's, in my exper[ience], I, this is a familiar pattern. * So I think I know what's going to happen next.	14:00	**For some reason I reassure myself—or her (that she is not alone?), by saying that I have seen this pattern before, which I have with other clients and that I can sometimes anticipate the upcoming transformation. But I pull back and remind her that I cannot fill in the blanks for her. Nor can she, for the brain.
212	C:	OK.		
213	P:	But, but, but why don't you just play with it. Stay with the green and, and take a look at it, and, and watch the green [traum ...], go past the green into...;* the brain is now trying to figure out what's inside.	14:15	

#	Speaker		Time	Notes
214	C:	It will let me go into the dark. Now it's the whole. Before it was this little tiny* thing out here.	14:30	*214-219. At the point where brain fully enters the traumatic pattern, it often seems as if the entire system, mind and body, is immersed in black. At this point, it is my understanding that the cellular awareness is accessed, in huge archipelagoes of connected cells or (molecule-)particles of cells throughout our mindbody. The proportionality of these island sequences might be as follows: some part of every cell in the body torques toward the left, in response to being hit by a car from the right, or some other similar pattern or conflicting patterns. In traumatic holding, the immobility message is sensed or communicated idiosyncratically throughout our being. Or better to say immobilization occurs at one level of every part, because the system continues to function except in this held place. Under the pressure of traumatic patterns seeking completion-resolution, this confounding, held place in the neurochemistry becomes the most important part for the brain until it is resolved, which may take years, decades, lifetimes. If not resolved, my guess is that many fatal diseases are directly related to early unresolved traumatic configurations. This is not a new insight.
215	P:	Right.		
216	C:	And when I, when I go into it, it [becomes]		
217	P:	It becomes the whole thing.		
218	C:	the whole thing.		

#		Utterance	Time	
219	P:	That. Now you're in the center of the trauma. You're closer to the center of the trauma.		219-232. I give an explanation and point of view from which to focus, including critically that of interest. What we are trying to do is get brain *interested* in those areas of its neurochemistry which are neurochemically troublesome yet cordoned off. The parallels with Kafkaland are direct. The first time we approach the black, the door is shut, the second time it is locked, the third time, the wall is sealed over, and a voice is responding," What door? There is no door here."
220	C:	Yeah [Yes.].		
221	P:	Can you see that?		
222	C:	Uh-huh [Yes.].		
223	P:	Isn't that interesting?		
224	C:	Yeah [Yes.].		
225	P:	Could you get used to that?		
226	C:	Uh-huh [Yes.].*	14:45	
227	P:	Yeah [Yes.], it's sort of interesting.		
228	C:	Yeah [Yes].		

#	Speaker	Utterance	Time	Notes
229	P:	You might see that that would be where you'd have to go		I explain how this process is repeatable; that in spite of its difficulty, she is in a different time, with different capacities, including those of interest, as opposed to freakout or crisis management or invocation of the trauma mechanism.
230	C:	To ge[t]....		
231	P:	in order to get out of one.		
232	C:	Yeah [I see.].		
233	P:	You know.		
234	C:	So I'm just surrounded by this like mud, like,		Black turns to brown, which I intuit means that the energy is no longer traumatically held in this place, but has transmuted into a more resilient (moving) brown, here implying energetic "bruise," but not energetic "hold."
235	P:	Yeah [OK.].		
236	C:	like chocolate.		
237	P:	Yeah. Is,		
238	C:	I'm surrounded by chocolate.		
239	P:	Is it brown or is it, is it* where's the...,	15:00	
240	C:	Yeah [Yes.].		
241	P:	or is it black?		

242	C:	It's not as black.		
243	P:	It's not as black.		
244	C:	Well, when you said that, it went to an, just a slightly lighter shade of brown.		
245	P:	Interesting.		
246	C:	An[d]...		
247	P:	It was black.*	15:15	
248	C:	When I first...		
249	P:	Can you find another section...?		
250	C:	When I first, when I first went into it, it was black. But now that I'm standing in it, it's not; it's like black. It's just, it's just like this close		250-257. Client has difficulty appraising the nature of the transformation—she is still in the middle of it. I try to indicate my presence and also give her permission to wave me off, as it were, to keep within her own preverbal, non-verbal process, yet to communicate to me when she can.
251	P:	Yeah [OK.].	15:30	
252	C:	I mean there's just like a tinge of,* I mean just, just....		
253	P:	OK, this is important. Stay with it. You're doing fine.		
254	C:	Yeah [Yes,], it's almost, it's, um....		

TRAUMA ENERGETICS

199

A SESSION

255	P:	Stay in that confusion and that difficulty appraising it and what.... Just stay with the colors. You don't have to describe it.*	15:45	
256	C:	Yeah [tentative "OK."].		
257	P:	And now I'll stay away from it; and you stay away from describing it.[???].[I won't say anything].		
258	C:	The bubble is starting to move this way [gesture]. *Humh.	16:00	
259	P:	Hmmh. What happened? You, if you're in the middle of a process, don't [speak]....		
260	C:	No, it's, it's just a, yuck; it's just that scene *that we were talking about before.	16:15	260-272. A narrative emerges, in an encapsulated (bubble) form, and the vision is clearer as brain appears to yield up the state of the art of dissociation within the trauma mechanism.
261	P:	Unh-hunh [OK.].		
262	C:	It's, it's, it's the adult standing around with the little child down[???drowned]there.		
263	P:	Right.		
264	C:	But it's* the, the bubble is allowing me to stay real far out of it.	16:30	
265	P:	Yup [Yes.].		
266	C:	I'm protected. I can lean up against the bubble almost like glass.		

267	P:	Yeap [Yes.].	
268	C:	And watch this, this trauma.	
269	P:	Your trauma. You're at the scene of whatever it is.		269, 271. I feel the need (whose?) to keep the process away from ego absconding with the energies connected with this resolution.
270	C:	Yeah [Yes.].	
271	P:	The trauma.	
272	C:	Yeah [Yes.]. * And that's now taken over the whole thing, and I'm watching from like, just this tiny little point way out here.	16:45	
273	P:	Yeah [Yes.]. * So you, you have to, at some point, you have to maybe almost leave the body, or it's similar to that or	17:00	I offer strategy to approximate the dissociation which trauma entails.
274	C:	Oh, yeah [yes.].		
275	P:	So you're, we're in a traumatic structure here. You can see it, that that's the way it looks.		275-279. We are here to learn about held-energy systems, even as we re-process them. As we do this, our doing is focused toward the goal of learning.
276	C:	Yeah [Yes.].		

277	P:	You, you fractionate, you separate out,* you put glass between it[t]. The mechanics of it, the architecture of it is very interesting.	17:15	Too many "you's" for my current understanding. This sounds very analytic to me, and hopefully, I would not do it this way now, I might say, "In my understanding," or "I think brain does this and this to render a recognizable perspective, so that we can return to this part of the lesson plan at a later time." This is a benchmark lesson. As I understand him and others, Levine conceives the trauma mechanism to engender a big bang phenomenon: a universal whole shatters into smaller integrities, held-energy systems, in order for the grander integrity to be maintained as a possibility. Yet brain appears to focus upon one "planetary system" then another, in the hope of bringing them all together into one sense of wholeness, where parts and connection add up into a "just right" sense, a neurochemical Eden of balance and integrity.
278	C:	Yeah [Yes.].		
279	P:	And, and totally understandable in order to to su[rvive], you know, allow the, the neurochemistry to survive.		279-294. Further underpinning and positioning. From this place in the chemistry, a new, deeper vision seems possible, taking the form of this insight.
280	C:	It's interesting. * I'm on a completely different place. When I saw this before, I was over here but looking down. I'm now not even in the room.	17:30	
281	P:	Umhm [OK.].		
282	C:	I'm looking in from a completely different point,* seeing people. Oh, it's almost like now that I'm looking over a grave.	17:45	
283	P:	Oh.		

284	C:	Oh, it's like there was a death in me at* that point or something.		
285	P:	Yes, something like that. Interesting.	18:00	**I think the black color of trauma reads like death, and may be coded in the same color as death, implying the same immobility, but it is not death, though it appears to mimic it. I remind her because seeing up-river a bit ahead of her, I sense we shall be entering a more difficult place, and she may need reminding about the difference between the present neurochemistry she is in (the trauma relating to the past), and the real present in which she does not have to again leave her body.
286	C:	Something really, like just said, "No more."		Describing, not experiencing the parameters of the energetic.
287	P:	No more. That I[???], I want to die.		I put in my two cents—is this supportive or merely trying to overcome my own painful awareness of a tradition of analytic cold turkey distancing?
288	C:	There's real powerful sadness. Now I,* some decision was made	18:15	288-290. Processing the trauma, the client now takes charge, knowing what the bubble is. She is now describing process, following the directions on the package as it were. Neither of us are doing anything but watching the completion process, or the setting up of the platform for viewing completion.
289	P:	Umum [OK].		
290	C:	a-against my parents, that they had allowed m[e], they had sent me to this. And that th-there[fore?] I can't trust again.		

#		Utterance	Time	Notes
291	P:	Yes. [???inaudible] You can't.... *	18:30	
292	C:	Yeah [Yes.]. And I floated in now.		
293	P:	You're coming back in.		
294	C:	I'm in the scene.		
295	P:	Yeap [Yes.].		
296	C:	I'm, I've moved just inside the bubble.		
297	P:	Right.		
298	C:	Um, and* floating.	18:45	
299	P:	Yeap [OK.]		
300	C:	Just seeing, it's almost like the, um, the child lying on the ground flashes between that and the gray.		300-312 Segments of the post-big-bang fractionation appear to be reassembled or juxtaposed.
301	P:	There we go.		
302	C:	It's like a flashing.		
303	P:	Wow.		
304	C:	And....		
305	P:	The brain is trying to work through the couple of, *-'s, there may be more than one sensation there.	19:00	I provide a strategy, tentatively, because we are exploring the reality together.
306	C:	Yeah [Yes.].		

#	Speaker	Utterance	Time	Commentary
307	P:	Or something. It's, it's probably, it's, it's a process.		The best I can do with what she is presenting. I confirm its reality and encourage her, I hope, to just watch it.
308	C:	Yeah [Yes,], it's not letting either one of them stick.		308-322. She is caught describing a relatively fast moving and complex energetic pattern and transferring it to language centers of brain. Unlike sportscasters, who have all their neuron calcium channeled from sensing to speaking before the game (they know the moves, plays, etc.), this client is describing something she has not seen before which heretofore she has been educated to experience as unimportant.
309	P:	Right.	19:15	
310	C:	And these people are just spectators now. Well,*		
311	P:	Umum [OK.].		
312	C:	they were both times.		
313	P:	Umum [OK.].		
314	C:	Now they're just, they're just, now it's kind of more. I see them again and the gray [grave???] moves* be[low], just below the surface. Just below the ground.	19:30	
315	P:	Interesting.		I respond with guidance on how to focus; we want the brain to get interested. I am not sure this is the best way, but it sort of works, over time. And again, the guidance reflects a specific, limited, and most powerful objective, namely to watch.

#			Time	
316	C:	The grave's below the ground now, and the, and the, the* child's there. And there's just a whole bunch of sorrow. And a lot of anger up here in this –		
317	P:	Yeah [Yes.].		
318	C:	And a lot of anger up here in this		
319	P:	Yeah [Yes.].*	19:45	
320	C:	entity.	20:00	**She describes the held-energy system as an entity. Every time we see such an entity, I read "system which needs dissolving." This is a goal consistent with what I perceive to be the erotic, mobile nature of life energy. The confusions about the nature of the energetic get expressed in the held-energy grid which infuses and structures our current understanding of sexuality (see Appendix). It does not surprise me when traditionally trained therapists apprehend the energetic through sexual energy and experiences, and so get caught in honoring that level of truth, and end up in bed with clients as the only way to access the energetic. My guess is that predominantly, they are attempting to complete their own traumatic patterns; yet they retraumatize themselves and their clients, because they are paradoxically caught in the narrative in movements which appear to disregard narrative by liberating them from cultural norms.
321	P:	Yep [Yes.]. I've got it.		
322	C:	In the scene it looks like the tape stops.		She is finding an appropriate analogy shorthand to tell me where she is.

#		Dialogue	Time	Commentary
323	P:	Yep [OK]. Who knows?*		
324	C:	Just to watch, or....something...	20:15	She continues.
325	P:	Just to watch, yeah. Maybe just to see something, just let brain scan. Until we can figure* out what to look at[???inaudible].*	20:30	I support her witnessing process amid the complexity of the energetic. It is not as if I want her to have a catharsis or anything demonstrably "releasey" (far from it). I believe feelings characterize energy at a different level from the one I am focusing on, and while they may play a part in the process, for the bulk of clients who have had a lot of experience with releasing or expressing feelings, their patterns have not changed. In these cases, some other approach must be devised. When a client has some feeling state ("I feel sad," for example, or starts to cry) as soon as seems appropriate or comfortable, I offer to "archive" the feelings, insights, or memories, as I direct her back to witnessing at the color level. There, it seems, brain gets the chance to finally solve the problem for good, not just to express it, and to retraumatize.
326	C:	There's just a desire to not watch this, not do *this, not. Just put it away.	20:45	We see her "resistance," only it is now out on the table where it is an experience she is not narratively immersed in; now brain may clarify and dissolve the pattern.
327	P:	Right.		
328	C:	Just, ah,		
329	P:	Had enough.		

TRAUMA ENERGETICS

A SESSION

330	C:	Yeah [Yes.].		
331	P:	Yeah [Yes.].		
332	C:	As I say that, it flashes, or it moves. *	21:00	She locates an interface between language and energy.
333	P:	Um-hum [Yes.].		
334	C:	Back out and then back again, and out and back in.		
335	P:	Uhm-hm [OK].		
336	C:	*There's also this thing going, "Come on, play out."	21:15	
337	P:	That's just come in?		I seem to be a backup witness, a recording stenographer.
338	C:	Uh-huh [Yes.].		
339	P:	All right, got something.		
340	C:	This thing going, "Come on."		
341	P:	That's the light [life???] energy coming back in. * Is it encouraging you to do something or just to complete something?	21:30	341-342. We are strategizing together, and the client is the primary reporter. I am sensing the pattern from her words as well as from the information I pick up skin to skin.
342	C:	Complete.		
343	P:	Isn't that interesting?		Again, the value of bringing brain to where it can be interested. Brain's interest, erotic, exploratory, and energetic, seems to stand against the neurochemistry which prohibits entering the black.

344	C:	Yeah [Yes.].		
345	P:	That's what the, you're looking straight at the energy there. Looking at something very deep there.		
346	C:	Yeah [Yes,], and it's been something that's been waiting for a long time.*	21:45	
347	P:	Yep. Um-hum [OK.].		
348	C:	Yup [Yes.].		
349	P:	Yeah [Yes.].		
350	C:	"Come on." Yeah.		
351	P:	So….		
352	C:	A total loss of, I don't know how to cross it.		
353	P:	Don't know what to do.		
354	C:	Yeah [Yes.].		
355	P:	Don't know what to do. So you're in the right place. This is, in this portion of the brain, you don't know what to do.*	22:00	355-356. We hover in the complexity of the chemistry, expressed by "Don't know what to do." This is where we want to be, not to push the situation beyond this immobility, and not to avoid it in other ways. These types of places are our focus. When brain witnesses them, it can reprogram this section of its chemistry.

356	C:	Um-um [No.].	
357	P:	In other portions you might, and probably you did. But this, well, this portion of the brain-mind, because you don't know, it's the most important one. What....	357-359. Here is a major tenet of this approach. ** There appear to be sections of the neurochemistry, and brain is always offering up the most difficult places for resolution; that seems to be its preoccupational task. Given the right (positive) platforms, it will force these problematic places forward with a mind-boggling rapidity. The movement is so fast, you think you are talking one second to the open self, the next second you are being offered an (acted out) traumatic pattern for solution.

In the midst of trauma, when the client experiences the black as saturatedly total, it is good to have set out a platform of understanding which says that there are other places in the system wherein functioning is not immobilized. Of course, that "insight" or framing doesn't matter to brain, which wants this "bad" place solved. And interestingly, the knowledge of other parts of well-functioning seem to be of no use at the center of the held-energy system. Brain has gotten into the middle of this and brain must get itself out. What I as facilitator offer is the platform of trust, equilibrium, and energetic connection through touch, which in fact sets brain to hunt in its attic for the patterns of stuck energy. |
| 358 | C: | And I can't even hardly hold onto the [a???] picture any more. | |
| 359 | P: | Yes, *it's tough. Is there any coloration, should we try the color? | 22:15 |

#			Time	
360	C:	Well, the picture is almost, I can't pull it back in if I try. E-everything went to this gray.* There's red.	22:30	She appears to understand the rubric of the energetics and is beginning to feel the chemical torques which keep her from getting the pattern distinct. She is like a fisher landing a big one, supported by a guide.
361	P:	Uhn-huh [OK.].*	22:45	
362	C:	It's like a, a was-, a whoosh,		
363	P:	It's now wash....		
364	C:	a moving,		
365	P:	Now it's....		
366	C:	a moving,		
367	P:	Yes,		
368	C:	moving.	23:00	
369	P:	This is, this is a, the brain is recomputing the information. You've had a glimpse. You're OK, you know.*		
370	C:	Unh-huh [Yes.].		
371	P:	You're in [Dallas]. [Chuckle.]		
372	C:	Uh-huh [Yes.].		

373	P:	And it will now go through [???] into the colors. Shall we, shall we e-enter one of the colors and see what we get?		
374	C:	Yeah [OK.].		
375	P:	Yeah [OK.]. OK. Let's do it. Let's go into the, * shall we try gray again?	23:15	
376	C:	Let's do gray.		
377	P:	Do you want to do that one? What are, what are the colors that are, are there?		
378	C:	Everything is a, like, there's this blue like wire, * neon wire kind of moving through, and,	23:30	
379	P:	Umhm [OK.].		
380	C:	and there's….		

381	P:	Is that new?	
		I don't know what particularly to say, so I sometimes revert to a stratagem. If I don't know, it usually means that the client is midprocess. My confusion is hers as well, and we need to deal with that to regain our focus and territory. One overall platform is relational, that I am a sharer in the process, that we are using her information and energetics as our primary data and concern. As her information has impact on me, I may comment on it to her, as part of the two person system we encompass. Part of that commentary may include defining statements that I am not penetrating her aura, or system, intentionally.	
		At strategic points in the session, I have reminded some victims of sexual abuse that I will not sexually abuse them even though I have told them before we work that I will not. And they would know from common sense that among other considerations, it would be retraumatizing, exploiting, not to mention the end of my career, if I were to do such a thing. Our collective viewpoint is that neither of us, client nor practitioner, violate or abuse her system energetically. We shift perspectives in order to focus on watching.	
382	C:	Uh-huh [Yes.]	
383	P:	Umhm [OK.] What else?	
384	C:	It's the, it's like, it's like* st-stuff being mixed together.	23:45

385	P:	Yes, this is an integrative process.*	23:45	The more she hangs out in the difficulty and the longer she stays there, the more familiar the brain appears to be with it; the colors, appropriately, lighten up. As brain gets accustomed to the situation, more relevant details show up for us to observe and respond to. In this process brain seems to need to see the complexity in its most held form before it can solve it in its own way. Over time, clients and I can begin to tell when we are facing the bottom line and when we are not. There is a begrudging tolerance for the client's going to the sidelines for a time out, especially when some new level of trust has been opened up by heading toward the black.
386	C:	And things are trying to [attach], except nothing knows where to attach.		If we were in analytic or meaning-centered (meaning-garnering) modes, we would spend days shooting off in that direction, including commentary on emotional attachments, early development, etc. While allowing those insights to show up, this technique does not consider that primary, even desirable information. The insights merely keep the status quo at the verbal, narrative level, and we never get to see the pattern change.
387	P:	Yeah, where...?		
388	C:	Where the, and there's some red all of a sudden.		**As the problem emerges increasingly into distinct energetic focus, and brain notes intensity—heat, anger, potential healing, whatever—the specific feeling or "meaning" is not central to the reworking at the color level for this *educational* process.** In contradistinction, the declaration of the feeling state (such as "I felt angry"), coupled with meaning or insight statements is considered desirable in *therapeutic* modalities.

#	Speaker		Time	
389	P:	Yeah [Yes.].		
390	C:	And when the red comes* in, it's almost like the red res[olves???], seems like to me going into my body or something.	24:00	390-391. It seems a major vector is changing, connected to dissociative process. This "mechanism" may have to change direction more than once until brain reads it in the proper order.
391	P:	Um-hum [OK.]. Um, are you going to resolve this at the body level do you think?		I ask a parameter-type question which in this case is not inappropriate, because the client responds with a direct answer. When the answer is not as forthcoming, then often I may say, "Erase that question."
392	C:	Uh, maybe. The reds, the red almost forces, where before I was seeing* it out here. The red makes me see it from in here.	24:15	The pattern appears inside something where before it had been outside. She seems to sense that as better.
393	P:	Yeah [Yes.].		
394	C:	And it's almost like it's all pushing down. Um, now,* the blue is on top of me.	24:30	The vector pressure described here may refer to a specific physical experience, such as being pushed down. The appearance of blue on top narratively suggests sky to me, or water, but my imagery association is a side order, not the main course.
395	P:	Um-hum [OK.].		
396	C:	It's just all this stuff's coming [in] this direction.		
397	P:	Different vector?		397-407. These are the kind of questions I find myself asking as we, client and practitioner, stay with the image.

398	C:	Yeah, everything is flowing* into me.	24:45
399	P:	Um-hum [OK.].	
400	C:	Almost like a lifeline.	
401	P:	Yeah [Yes.].	
402	C:	The lifeline is trying to be reassuring* or something.	25:00
403	P:	It's a reassuring color and a reassuring energy.	
404	C:	Uh-huh [Yes.].	
405	P:	Yuh [OK.].	
406	C:	But it's forcing, there's this like	
407	P:	There's a forced quality to it.	
408	C:	You have to go up into the black. You have to.... *	25:15	408-439. That she goes into the black seems different from the ordinary experience of black, namely that it is forbidden, and that there would be an energetic pushing away (resistance) to that. Sometimes the black seems as if it were a comfort or refuge to the client, in which case I assume there are more difficult layers ahead. Here she notes some pressure —having to go up into the black. I sense this to be a "life pattern," if you will, of considerable importance.

| 409 | P: | Umum [Thoughtful.] So maybe this is a kind of near-death experience of some sort. | I am trying to get oriented here, as well as to set some focusing parameter, in the face of the complex neurochemical flux. I intuit that the red appearing in the black indicates we have unlocked the puzzle a bit, and so more information (not narrative) will be forthcoming. Using this approach, narrative is not information; it conveys the energetic but it confounds when read as important. An equivalent metaphor might be to take the label and advertising about Coca-Cola to be prior in importance to its sensate experience. |
| | | | My experience with sexually-abused incest victims (not the case here) suggests that there is endless blaming and abusive assumption of responsibility on the part of the victim, and inwardly, probably, with the perpetrator, as we hold on to the narrative. There are critical points where the child will take on the abusing parent's energy pattern out of love, desire to heal, etc., and then find that the patterns are not being correctly discerned within their combined system. Brain is not particularly reassured by reminding the victim that they were not to blame nor that they thought they were. The pattern seems held at some auric, subtle body level or an equivalent and thus must resolve energetically, not narratively. It is the relationship of the energetic to the narrative, occurring at the crux of sexuality, where energy and movement interact in confounding ways, which appears more difficult for brain than the details of the abuse. (*Continued next cell*). |

#	Speaker		Time	Commentary
410	C:	Yeah, and		*(Continued from above cell)*. It seems there must be some way for the client(-child) to see into the problem which the perpetrating parent has with its parent before the healing occurs. Staying with the victimhood of the child has not worked with the clients I have seen. Ultimately clarifying the narrative does not increase the informational mastery or reduce the toxicity, for it does not expose the original desire to connect energetically with and to heal the parent's held-energy system.
411	P:	That you have		
412	C:	And		
413	P:	There emotional, actually physical or something. You drop out of a tree or something as a child, or something happened.*	25:30	My syntax deserts me as I stumble to the idea, and find myself reapproaching the true narrative.
414	C:	No, I went under a boat. Wow! That's what that forcing is. It's the bottom of the boat..		The client becomes very certain here, and the story emerges and has a clarity to it which conveys the traumatic *energetic* elaboration which the client is following. The drama and the accuracy of the commentary seems fine enough to me. Brain unlocks the puzzle if you follow the energy pattern, even as the feelings and story are expressed. It is the loss of this connection with the energy which the trauma mechanism sets in which appears of ultimate confoundment to brain, not the narrative occasion which sets it in place (I was going to write "sets it in motion," but of course that is not what it is doing).
415	P:	Umm.		

416	C:	When I was real little, I fell off that. Oh, I remember. It was a big black boat.*	25:45	
417	P:	Yup [Yes.].		
418	C:	And I went under the boat and hit, my head hit, kept, my head, like, hit the bottom of the boat.		
419	P:	Um-hum [OK.].		
420	C:	And then something grabbed me and threw me out the side of the boat*		420-438. Brain seems to be integrating the new information, with insight summary-type statements typical of this phase of integration of the new information which has been processed. While I respect this new "evidence," I do not consider it significant to the mobilization process, which appears to require that we stay with the energetic.

| 421 | P: | Umhum [OK]. | 421–425. All of these insights would be fine for analysts to hang out with for decades, but change can be evoked at an alternate level, and we must return to that. ** I think this shift in focus distinguishes this approach from others, including energy-related modalities like bioenergetics, neurolinguistic programming, rebirthing, and breathing techniques. They are often focusing upon the denser narratives of the body structure (as are Rolfers), at factors like breathing and muscular tonus. As a result, they induce or initiate gross motor responses into these nexuses of held energy, blasting them, or substituting, overlaying, rather than watching the held energy unlock itself. In some situations, this latter witnessing function seems to be the only answer brain is satisfied with because the information it contains is then integrated by the brain at multiple, complex neurochemical levels beyond conscious imagining. Even though they access new material by their attenuated modalities, bioenergetic exercises, structural integrations, religious insights, and healing touch, they may retraumatize at every point, and so at some critical level the deepest patterns never change. This strategy puts the primacy on staying with the subtle energetic, which means that in the session, the client does not move very much. If they do, it is as an act of integrating kinesthetically with the energetic which has been rediscovered or witnessed for the first time. In this sense this approach holds more kinship with traditional analytic insights, which intuit that the energetic needs some "analytic" distancing to be able to process held energy. Paradoxically, by keeping at a verbal level, a verbal analytic approach may prolong the trauma (*Continued next cell*). |

422	C:	underwater.	*(Continued from above cell).* by not having any way to focus upon the energetic and bring brain to focus. By staying in the narrative levels of emotion, and verbal discourse, the analyst may direct attention from the subtle body and cellular interface levels which ultimately hold the traumatic patterning. One reason for long and unsatisfying analyses?
423	P:	Wow!	
424	C:	I left my body then, too. And I had,* something grabbed me and made me go back into my body.	26:00
425	P:	Um-hum [OK]. You were all ready to leave.	
426	C:	Oh. And I wanted* to.	26:15
427	P:	Sure.	
428	C:	I wanted to leave.	
429	P:	[Inaudible. Good God.???]	
430	C:	I was angry at, I was being forced to get back into life.	
431	P:	Yeah [Yes.].	

432	C:	I didn't want to be in life. I wanted to go ahead and leave.* I created that to leave. And they wouldn't let me leave.** Wow! I created it over and over again. God, as a little kid I didn't want to be here.	26:45
433	P:	Humhm [OK.].	
434	C:	I fell, and I kept doing it with boats. I've always fallen off boats. * I wanted to leave. And there was this power that kept saying, with anger almost, "No," and, "Stop doing it."	27:00
435	P:	Um-hum [OK.].*	27:15
436	C:	Then I had to tread water. That's what that, somehow this....*	27:30
437	P:	The darker force over, in the light?	
438	C:	Well, I'm out here* in the water, and I feel like I'm just treading water.	27:45
439	P:	Yep [Yes.].	
440	C:	Just constantly treading water, trying to keep my head up.	
441	P:	Yep [Yes.].	
442	C:	And when I get tired, oh, my neck hurts in back real bad.	
443	P:	Stay in that. *Just let that, you know, we'll put that on the shelf. Put the pain of that on th[e], you know....	28:00
444	C:	Yeah [OK.].	

445	P:	Don't. You stay in the energy and let the insights come forward.	
446	C:	I was just like, * over here [gesture] is a, what are those things, a whirlpool, like	28:15	446-447. A new set of vectors appear in the sequence, and the chemistry reworks. At a subtle energy level, some people characterize whirlpool shapes as chakra structures (Bruyere) which can get blocked. Here this client follows the chemical lead and seems to be examining an old sequence for the first time, perhaps because brain knows, for the first time in this phase of the chemistry, that she is no longer at risk.
447	P:	Uhmhm [OK.].		
448	C:	that pulls you down under the water.		
449	P:	Yep [Yes.].		
450	C:	Yes. * There's like Mom's and Dad's shit.	28:30	

451	P:	Good. It's their pattern.	At this level she can see how some of the pattern is not hers, but "her parents". This kind of differentiation is processed at an energetic, not an insight or so-called boundary level. It is based upon something beyond ideas, because it has an observational quality, focusing on the energetic, not even the relational. The insight would seem to be based upon a reality which can be honored, instead of disembodied psychodynamic commentary, all of which may be true at some level, but which does not change the pattern which is bothering brain, in a "language" which brain understands, with a syntax which respects brain's process. The recognition of where the pattern comes from, back into the second, or third generation, can be intuited from this energetic level. The brain can usually give up the pattern when it reaches the, say, grandparental lineage. A similar phenomenon occurs in the apprehension that Jesus is born of a Virgin Mary, who herself must have been born of a virgin (St. Anne). The perpetrating parent must be seen as a child who endured similar perpetrations from its parents.
452	C:	Yes. And I've been out here treading water, doing everything I can to not pull into that.	A spatial and dramatized statement of what she has been doing in this portion of the chemistry ever since the accident, maybe before. The key issue here is the varied direction of the conflicting vectors, all of which, it is my experience, are expressed in compressed molecular, cellular, muscle, and structural "stress" patterns.
453	P:	Yes.	

454	C:	And I would get tired and just decide I just don't want to do this*	28:45	
455	P:	Umhum [OK.].		
456	C:	and go over the side of the boat.		
457	P:	Hmm.		
458	C:	There's this thing * saying, "No, go ahead and go down the..."	29:00	
459	P:	Down the chute or something. Down the,		I start with the cliché, the first thing that occurs, as I try to fill in the blanks for her. It is interesting that now I tell the clients that may fill in the blanks by finishing their sentences, and that if I make a mistake, they should correct me. As they confront the interface between the energetic and language, it seems all right, even preferable, if they speak in fragments, in whatever ways they do. We follow their process and enable us both to get out of the speech functions of the brain, to allow the brain its own process at a different and usually abandoned level. I intuitively return to the energetic idea of vortex, rather than a literal situation. Each time the literality occurs (in a kind of fundamentalist strategy), the static nature of the imagery is worked with until there is movement and reengagement with the energetic levels. For the client to do this while using words is a bit of an acquired taste (and skill).
460	C:	Down that, yeah,		

TRAUMA ENERGETICS

A SESSION

461	P:	that,		
462	C:	that chute.		
463	P:	that vortex.		
464	C:	It is a vortex, a very powerful vortex.		
465	P:	Yes.*	29:15	
466	C:	It's....		
467	P:	Tha.... Are you going to do it?		
468	C:	Yeah, here we go.		
469	P:	OK, here we go. Is there a color to it?		
470	C:	Yeah, it's a, um, an angry blue.		
471	P:	Yes. Yes. Yeah.		
472	C:	And, and as, as* I move towards it, all this blackness follows me	29:30	
473	P:	Hmm.		
474	C:	down into this vortex. But then it's not very long. * As soon as I go into it, it's like going into a slide,	29:45	
475	P:	Hmhm [OK.].		

				To me the oil indicates some movement, some flexibility but not necessarily some core pattern completed.
476	C:		and I'm back in the darkness. It's like I see, the blackness follows me. And I go, [a]nd I'm just surrounded by oil.	
477	P:		There you go.	
478	C:	30:00	*Surrounded by this blackness. Just totally.	She is immersed in the black, an archipelago of cellular and molecular holding throughout the mindbody.
479	P:		So you're in the, in [the].... Whose blackness are you in at this point? Is it theirs or yours?	Not sure of this—but I want to clarify the boundary issues here, to line up the perspective. This is a usual question I find myself asking, but less now than before. I used to employ it in an effort to force the bud of recognition that in fact, the client has taken on the energetic of the parents, or their traumatic situation, whatever, which did not belong with the child. In a way, I think I was pushing this "focus" because I knew the boundary issues it contained involved deep disturbance, not just because of the violations. Apparently, the information contained in the violations is more important than the narrative through which it is expressed. Entire cultural lineages of abuse thus may be contained in the patterns perpetrated upon victims by victims. The client can see this and for the first time, shift these patterns and dissolve them, as the information is absorbed and integrated. There is no putting off, or setting aside of these patterns.

#	Speaker	Text	Time	Annotation
480	C:	I think it's mine now.		480–497. We can see how the pattern was absorbed, the history of it, which I think is more interesting than its so-called substance. The way it is taken on "molecularly" suggests a perspective from which to watch the change. If there is no "platform" from which to witness this reworking, I intuit that brain has difficulty "catching its breath," before immersing into the process again.
481	P:	It's yours now. Was it theirs?	30:15	
482	C:	Yeah, the black;* I slid into it. I was sliding into their stuff.		
483	P:	Right.		
484	C:	But as soon as I entered that oil, it's mine.		
485	P:	It's yours. Interesting.		
486	C:	And....		
487	P:	It's a critical place. Isn't that an interesting place?		
488	C:	Wow! Yeah [Yes.]. I had to go through theirs * to get into mine.	30:30	
489	P:	Yeah [Yes.].		
490	C:	And it's just this, it's just, it's, it's black oil.		
491	P:	Great.		
492	C:	It, and it's * a, and it's all encompassing. It's, you know,	30:45	

493	P:	Hmhuhm [OK.]		Brain processes the stress. The client appears on the way to taking out major traumatic sequence here at a very fundamental level. Our mindbody tells us where we are.
494	C:	it's, it's the, leaks into the pores.		
495	P:	Gets into the cells.		
496	C:	Yes.		
497	P:	Gets in the cellular level. So this is your cellular memory?*	31:00	
498	C:	Yes.		
499	P:	And you've taken it on.		
500	C:	The only thing, it's like the only thing that hasn't is I've been able to keep my head up.		500-501. A major dynamic is being identified, with client's chronic neck tension.
501	P:	Yeah [Yes.]. Yeah.		
502	C:	But everything else is completely surrounded in this, there's just a little bubble*	31:15	502-503. The bubble recurs, this time connected to the body situation, in a better alignment, or at least more distinctly than when it first occurred. The bubble has realigned around the head, probably commenting upon a kind of movement of a drowning person.
503	P:	Um-hum [OK.].		
504	C:	around my head.		

#	Sp.	Text	Time	Commentary
505	P:	Right. From this point of view, what needs to happen?		**A question of strategy—critical to bring brain into a consideration of options which in the rush of the trauma, it doesn't experience time to process at some gross level. Of course we can propose that it processes everything on some level because it survives.**
506	C:	I'd like to get out of the oil. (Laughter.)*	31:30	**A relief. We both find this funny.**
507	P:	(Laughter.)		
508	C:	(Laughter.) I don't think that that's an option.		
509	P:	(Laughter.) I don't either. (Laughter.) I, ah, isn't that funny?		
510	C:	Nothing changed when I said it, but I very much....		**510-527. Again, language is expected to transform, but it doesn't. Only to a certain degree, we leverage ourselves into transformations through language and its disciplines. But then brain and the energetic appear to revolt. And crucially, in the held-energy system, brain seems to need to work through the problem in the energetic, "independently" of language.**
511	P:	(Laughter.) Well, that's, I think that's brain's thought, is		
512	C:	(Laughter.)		
513	P:	"Let's get out of here."		
514	C:	Let's get out of here.*	31:45	
515	P:	Yeah [Yes.], but interesting. Is the black the black has some oily qualities,		

516	C:	Yeah [Yes.].		
517	P:	doesn't it?		
518	C:	Yeah [Yes.], it's really oily.		
519	P:	Yeah [Yes.].		
520	C:	It's real thick.		
521	P:	Yeah [OK.].		
522	C:	And not oil like, oil like what comes out of the ground, * oil.	32:00	
523	P:	Oil.		
524	C:	Or like dirty car engine oil.		
525	P:	Yes, right. Right. It's a muck.		
526	C:	Yeah [Yes.]. And somehow I'm moving off to the left now.		We see some shift, perhaps tracing an original movement or configuration, then by line 534, we are in a new sequence.
527	P:	Umum [OK.]		
528	C:	*But nothing happened. I'm just floating in the muck to the left	32:15	
529	P:	Yeah [OK.].		

#	Spk	Utterance	Time	Commentary
530	C:	for some reason.		
531	P:	Yep [OK].		
532	C:	like it, like there's a, there's a way to get to the surface.		
533	P:	Um-hum [OK].		
534	C:	But I'm not so sure I want to surf[ace]. You know, it's kind of like, * "No, no, no, stay down in here in the muck."	32:45	A new vector appears.
535	P:	Well, let's stay down here in the muck for a bit. I'm, I'm, I'm happy.		535-536. I joke, also intuitively state difference between her and me.
536	C:	I'm glad you are. (Laughter.)		We both joke over a desperate situation. Brain appears not cognizant in this place that it is free yet, that it is in a different time and place. There is no hypnosis here. We can make diversions, side comments, then return to the difficult material.
537	P:	(Laughter.) I don't think this bothers me as much as it does you. No, I'm picking it up, some of it. *	33:00	Our strategy is that the infant picks up other people's held-energy systems and has to learn that it can cope with these. But the original movement is an act of love, of erotic caring: "Let me help." Repeatedly, I witness an energy that takes on the sins of the world, if you will. This energy has been identified variously with Christ, or Buddha energy, something everyone has, but does not always sense. I offer a locator to indicate the concern—but only as a kind of workman's concern for the factors which will get us through this situation. As I close the sessions, I spend a great deal of time negotiating the separation to make sure it is clean and clear.

538	C:	Oh, OK.		
539	P:	There are a couple of things that interest me. One is the, is the division at the neck. I'm wondering if you, what would happen if you, if you		
540	C:	Yeah [Yes,], I couldn't breathe [above???].		
541	P:	You couldn't breathe.		
542	C:	Yeah [Yes,], it's all of a sudden suffocating. *Just the thought of, of taking that bubble off is th' total suffocation	33:15	The impact of the trauma is sensed, and we negotiate.
543	P:	Suffoca....		
544	C:	by this muck.		
545	P:	Yes. Yeah. So* let's see if we can under[stand]. Let's, let's, rather than, that's maybe another step, but not something we need to do now. *I mean that might be the next step of the, of the trauma which	33:45	
546	C:	Un-hunh [OK.].		
547	P:	you'll have to, you know, at some point you'll be able to tolerate that.		
548	C:	Uh-huh [Yes.].		

TRAUMA ENERGETICS

A SESSION

549	P:	But I don't think right now. The brain is saying, "Well, that's not, not such a great idea." So let's order, let's go in the order that it's, * t's presenting and see if we can do a microscopic view of one of the molecules that are there [??], and see if we can, we may, if, because of the magnitude of it, we might not be able to understand. *	34:00	** This is a hallmark of this technique, or mindset, that our awareness, whatever that is, can go to any place in the body, at any level of magnification. Here the client takes it up as her own tool. If brain decodes the smallest unit, then it can extrapolate to and resolve the larger experience. This approach might be useful for approaching systemic disorders, including cancer and immune disorders.
550	C:	Yeah, we can get to a little, we can see little drops.		
551	P:	You can?		
552	C:	I mean I can, I can make everything enlarged. *	34:15	
553	P:	Right.		
554	C:	So I can get to these little drops		
555	P:	That's it. There you go.		
556	C:	that are surrounded by.... But, oh, there we go. I can see the little, a little ball*	34:30	
557	P:	There, there you go.		
558	C:	drop.		
559	P:	There you go. There you go. If we understand one, the brain, the genius of the brain is able to extrapolate the entire, through		
560	C:	Unh-huh [OK.].		

561	P:	the whole body in a relatively short time. But it doesn't understand * this oil	34:45	
562	C:	Uhn-huh [No.].		
563	P:	at a molecular level, so let's go down there and see.		
564	C:	It's real. It's just like water. I mean oil.		564-573. Brain reevaluates the information at this new level.
565	P:	It's like oil?		
566	C:	Yeah [Yes.].		
567	P:	Is it shiny, * is the molecule? [Is it] shin[y]?	35:00	
568	C:	It's, it's just like a raindrop. I mean it moves and,* uh, you can put your hand through it and be empty [???inaudible].	35:15	
569	P:	Very good. So we're still in that sort of all pervasive, we're at cellular level here.		
570	C:	But		
571	P:	So....		
572	C:	it was still		
573	P:	It's still oil.		
574	C:	Uh-huh [Yes.].		

#	Speaker	Dialogue	Time	Commentary
575	P:	*At the molecular level, are you viewing one of the molecules? Or one of the particles? We may not be at the molecular level. But you've, at least you've reduced it	35:30	Currently, I think it misleading to call them molecules. I call them particles and say that I believe that we may be at a molecular level here, or a cellular level, depending upon the way the information is emerging or the sense in the client mindbody that such focus evokes. Often, when something resolves at this level, a stress pattern is reduced, which is perceived at the cellular level as a less tense and compressed, more open sensation.
576	C:	Unhha [Yes.].		
577	P:	to a single particle.		
578	C:	Uh-huh [Yes.]. Uh-huh [Yes.].		
579	P:	As you look at it, what needs to happen?*	35:45	When the particle is reduced to manageable size, then brain can be asked what to do. If there is real consternation, then one choice is to try to go into the particle and check out the terrain, or to enter the color of the particle and find a sub-level of magnification.
580	C:	[It] needs to be, something needs to be added to it * so that it dissolves or dissipates or....	36:00	At last brain appears to perceive what needs to be done. In the stunning impact of trauma neurochemistry, often brain seems at a loss to realize that anything can be done, or that the things it has tried in fact are unsuccessful. In the case of addictions, the sense of failure or impasse at this kind of interface may be profound and unassailable, especially if processed only by verbal insight and emotional, expressive means.
581	P:	Uhm-hum [OK]. Have you understood that before?		

#			Time	
582	C:	Um-um [No.].		
583	P:	That's a, we're changing a chemistry right in front of your eyes.		583-608. Brain reworks the new information, reporting its process in the form of an insight, in a pragmatic, functional way. On some level, we intuit that the sequence is actually occurring as she talks. She can see it and describe her experience.
584	C:	Yeah [OK.].		
585	P:	Isn't that fun?		
586	C:	It's like soap needs to be added.		
587	P:	Yeah [OK.]. Yeah. Something to* dissolve it. When it's dissolved, what will happen?	36:15	
588	C:	[I] can't get on it [me???there???]*.	36:30	
589	P:	Yeah [OK.]. Hang out with that. It doesn't, you know, it doesn't, you sort of, [resolve???hold] that way. If it dissolves, what's going to happen?		
590	C:	It will go away.		
591	P:	*It will go away. How will it go away?	36:45	
592	C:	Just changes.		
593	P:	It will change?		

594	C:	It just, [it'll] is[???] no longer be the same. Um,* I think it just goes away.*	37:00
595	P:	Right. Will it flush out, or will it just be transformed?	
596	C:	No, just trans[formed]. It looks like it goes from oil base* to just, um, light as a cloud kind of steam.	37:15
597	P:	It's, it's going to turn into a vapor?	
598	C:	Yeah [Yes.].	
599	P:	And then it will be, whatever toxicities are in it will....	
600	C:	Just be, just float out.*	37:30
601	P:	Just pulled [float???] out.	
602	C:	And it keeps doing it [Laughter.] Over and over.	
603	P:	[Laughter.]	
604	C:	I say it, it becomes a ball.	
605	P:	Yes.	
606	C:	Something drops on it, and it dissolves and, and lifts* and goes. And then it does it again.	37:45

#			
607	P:	Yes. So we're in a, in a confessional-sin-forgiveness pattern here.	Brain may not have gone to the bottom of the pattern and so hovers in what I describe using religious terms, here in the wrong order, namely the cycle where we "sin," confess, get forgiven, and then repeat the sin, confess, etc.—a never-ending loop until we finally see the point of origin of the addictive pattern and conclude the entire sequence. As addictive pattern and Twelve Steppers know very well, premature "forgiveness" here can be a sustainer of addictive process, not a conclusion of it. I am not sure if I would introduce theological strategies without preparation at the beginning. Some clients are frightened by them; others welcome the commentary and clarification of these older strategies from the energetic point of view.
608	C:	Yes.	
609	P:	It's, you know, it's going in and out. But it isn't replace.... What shall, can we get rid of the whole pattern?	609-610. I propose this strategy, which may be a possibility (hope) which has not been envisionable up to now. It is as if brain is deserted or isolated from a sense of possibility when the pressure to complete the held-energy system is of such magnitude.
610	C:	(Laughter.)* Uh. We[ll], ye[ah]. Um.	38:00
611	P:	What, what does brain think? Or does it know what to do?	

#	Speaker	Dialogue	Time	Notes
612	C:	No.		Brain appears not to know what to do. There is no judgment here, only observation. And with that, perhaps right action in the form of witnessing the process. We are not at the bottom of the pattern which has appeared as a loop, over and over.
613	P:	Brain doesn't know what to do with this.		
614	C:	It's just trying		
615	P:	It's trying		
616	C:	out		
617	P:	out, (Laughter.) it's trying out putting soap on it. (Laughter.) It's		
618	C:	Yeah, it's trying....		
619	P:	It's turning into a vapor.		
620	C:	Yeah [Yes.].*	38:15	
621	P:	It still doesn't get it out.		
622	C:	Unh-hunh [No.].		
623	P:	OK.		

#		Text	Time	
624	C:	No, it's because I've got this little dot, that there's these, it's like every time there's more dots to replace the little dot.		624-625. This hydra-like phenomenon suggests we have brought some sequence forward, *i.e.*, set it in motion or recognized it as having been happening for a long time. It involves brain reworking the relationship between one and many, only we have not approached it in a manner which unlocks the information in the order brain can handle it. Again, the lesson is to follow the directions on the package. Attempts to get some pattern out which brain experiences as undesirable seem not to work if they are hatcheted, smashed, abandoned, particle-ized, shunted off, whatever. In order to self-dissolve (self-crumble) they must be witnessed and understood at this energetic level. This process is essentially described in Sophocles' *Oedipus at Colonus*.
625	P:	Yeah, right, exactly. There's some behind the earlier. [???]*	38:30	
626	C:	That flashed on snails or something.		
627	P:	Snails?		
628	C:	Um, no matter what you put out there,		628-634. The hydra process.
629	P:	Yeah.		
630	C:	there will still be more snails.		
631	P:	Snails. * They'll still be more snails, yes, to deal with. [That's???] perfect[???].	38:45	

632	C:	(Laughter.)	
633	P:	This is ma-, this is maddening.	633. I speak for both of us. 633-657. We reconfigure, re-strategize. We speak about brain, trying to find the originating point of chemistry (Levine's *To*) where brain may openly confront the information contained in the held-energy system.
634	C:	Yeah, it's going, there's just, there's just, there's so much of it.	
635	P:	Right. Let's figure another way of doing, going, ... *	39:00
636	C:	Uh-huh [OK].	
637	P:	You've got the scenario. It's a little uncertain, isn't it?	
638	C:	Uh-huh [Yes.].	
639	P:	We sort of know. But brain really doesn't know. So let's go back to the place where we don't know what the hell to do with this.	
640	C:	Yeah [OK].	
641	P:	Go back into the chemistry of that.	
642	C:	OK.	
643	P:	*Staying in that portion. Now you, how [are???] you doing?	39:15

644	C:	Uh-huuh [somewhat uncertain]. Yeah, and when you said that, it,[???] it was short of leaving* it.	39:30	We are in some real confusion, but rather than overlook it, we are witnessing it with some interest, even, ultimately, enthusiasm.
645	P:	Yeah [OK.].		
646	C:	That's been the most recent pattern.		
647	P:	Yeah [OK.]. You just walk away, then.		
648	C:	Throw it off, you have to die. You have to be....		Here is one of the "assumptions" of defeat. The pattern is too much.
649	P:	You have to die.		
650	C:	I, to leave it.		
651	P:	To leave that.* All right. So 't, so it, so, talk.	39:45	** I want to hear in addition to the processing which she is undergoing preverbally. It is a judgment call when to do this and when not. Ultimately, a rhythm or pace is set between practitioner and client so that these overlapping interfaces do not destroy the moment of witnessing, which neither client nor practitioner possess; neither of us "do" anything.
652	C:	I'm in the midst[???] of so much of it		
653	P:	Isn't that something?		I support her ability to sustain focus in the complexity and chaos.

654	C:	that, that, that was part of, that connects into the drowning pattern. Now, it's just the water is the same thing as the oil in a way.*	40:00	Further connection, leading to a partial equalizing of oil and water.
655	P:	Um-hum [OK].		
656	C:	There's so much of it that, you know, just leave.		
657	P:	Just leave.		
658	C:	Yeah [Yes.].		
659	P:	Yeah [OK]. So this is a [the] real part of the drowning,		
660	C:	Yeah [Yes.]		
661	P:	drowning episode.		
662	C:	Yeah [Yes.].		
663	P:	*Take a look at the molecule again, if you've got it.	40:15	Again, I now do not like to delineate it as a molecule. It is too determinate to label it molecule, though I think that is the appropriate scale to be considering here, and to encourage the client to experience, for I believe the stress pattern can manifest at that level.
664	C:	Well, it's changing to be a little.... It, it's now coming back sort of to the water. * Instead of being black, it's more of a blue-green.	40:30	A beginning of change, but not secure. I sense we need to go back to the black.

665	P:	Um-hum [OK]. Is that a development or a, am avoidance, would you say? In other words, are we heading deeper into a resolution of the trauma or are we, is...?		
666	C:	*Pulling out of it.	40:45	
667	P:	We're pulling out of it. So let's go back to the black and see if we can get back		667-668. We go back into black as a choice, as a place to go, not experiencing the shielding, resistant power of the black
668	C:	OK.		
669	P:	to the oil. So let's not desert this part[icle]-		
670	C:	Yeah [OK].		
671	P:	-molecule. It's growing if we do[???]		
672	C:	OK. I'm there.		
673	P:	Are we there? Let's just....**	41:15	
674	C:	It's almost like a talking bubble.		A clarification here.
675	P:	Um-hum [OK]. It's a bubble now? It's not just a droplet?		675-687. Further clarification; brain may elaborate with combinations. This is the third time we have seen bubble, but it now combines with the oil, and with the head-neck, as in talking bubble.
676	C:	Yeah [Yes.]		

#		Utterance	Time	Notes
677	P:	Aha! * How did it get that? Is that just a transformation?	41:30	
678	C:	It's,		
679	P:	Is that chemical?		
680	C:	it, it was real globby [blobby???].		
681	P:	Yeah [OK.], it was kind of a thick mass [???]		
682	C:	And now it's more—it's the same color.		
683	P:	Um-hum [OK.].		
684	C:	But it's more of a bubble.*	41:45	
685	P:	So it's changing?		
686	C:	Yeah [Yes.].		
687	P:	So let's play with it a bit more. Stay with the idea that we don't know. It's, it's a talking bubble?		Decision to play with the situation, teasing it apart.
688	C:	No, well, it just kinda flashed on, um, like a soap bubble.		Soap and oil indicate a new combination, perhaps taking oil out.
689	P:	*Yep [OK.].	42:00	
690	C:	You know, or something.		
691	P:	So it's become, there's something about soap bubble and something about oil.		

692	C:	Yeah [Yes.].		
693	P:	And we're not sure. It's becoming a soap, soap bubble now in the, in the latest transformation.		
694	C:	Yeah [Yes.], it's still black, but it's,*	42:15	
695	P:	It's still black.		
696	C:	it's, it's trying to turn to white.		
697	P:	Yes. Yeah, yeah.		
698	C:	It's trying to,		
699	P:	Isn't that interesting?		
700	C:	it's trying to go from this oil to this [gesture].		
701	P:	Yeah [Yes.]. Stay, stay, stay, don't desert it. Stay in the impossibility* of it. Go back as close as you can to the place where it's oil and it doesn't move. It just, it won't come out.	42:30	I urge her to keep the focus where it is most difficult, where the immobility is most distinct. If this urging has intentionality, it is different from trying to "do" something, in the usual sense; it is a different kind of focusing energy that the client is used to in this place in the chemistry.
702	C:	OK, yeah [yes].		
703	P:	Do you know what I'm saying?		
704	C:	Uh-huh [Yes.].		

TRAUMA ENERGETICS

A SESSION

#		Dialogue	Time	Notes
705	P:	Really give your.... Every time we'll do* that we're going to get, we'll get a change. If we want to stay with the change, we've got to stay with the original situation.	42:45	705-706. **This is a reiterative explanation as to why we are going into the black. It is the old "the way out is by going through" strategy, but at a neurochemical level.
706	C:	OK. It's almost like I have to hold on.*	43:00	
707	P:	Yes, to do that?		
708	C:	Yeah [Yes.]		
709	P:	Yeah [Yes,], you say hold on. It would be nice if it could let go –.[don't have to hold on].*	43:15	
710	C:	*[???]The bubble wants, the black is becoming more of a shape of a rectangle, box. *	43:45	The energy appears to have some containing, perhaps rational qualities to it. Here the direction of the movement is of interest. Are we going toward or away from the center of the held-energy system? I include the client in the strategizing about this. Perhaps one way to tell if it is closer, and not a (defense) is that the energy is denser.
711	P:	There we go. Yes. Yup. You're seeing, I think, a sub-, you know, a sub-level of what it appeared to be. Is it, is it denser?		
712	C:	Uh-huh [Yes.]		
713	P:	Neat.* We're, we're closer to the core. This is closer to the core now, whatever that is.	44:00	
714	C:	Uh-huh [Yes.]		
715	P:	Does that feel right?		

#	Sp.	Text	Time	Notes
716	C:	Uh-huh [Yes.].		
717	P:	Isn't that interesting?		
718	C:	Yeah [Yes.].	44:15	
719	P:	So it's, it's a box?*		
720	C:	It, it started out just a square. Now it's like a black cedar box.		Cedar (*see there*, a side order of pun?) the oil becomes a box and is now beginning to become more organic, more resembling a tree. As I hear *tree*, I intuit we may be heading into a level of spinal (meningeal?) trauma patterning here, though the structure I think we may be looking at may not be that. What is important is to stay with the brain process as it locates itself, and then as the chemistry changes, we see where the relaxation, or twitch, or spasm occurs. Many clients report chronic patterns activated from these color forms, and watch them "dissolve," an odd and often new experience of direct "healing."
721	P:	There we go.		721-736. Brain works out permutations on the pattern.
722	C:	That can open.		
723	P:	That can open. It has a lid?*	44:30	
724	C:	Well, all it is is a lid of a box.		
725	P:	A lid of[???] a box.		

#			Time	Commentary
726	C:	And anger.*	44:45	Client proposes a feeling state, and I remind her to keep the focus at the energy level by underscoring that the feeling state can be considered a chemistry. I am not concerned with emotional discharge and its resultant disorientation—it is, within my current understanding, just not significant information. When true change is being processed, I find clients not in the upheaval of emotion (not to say that emotion does not have a part to play somewhere), but observational, quiet, and more awefull.
727	P:	Uhm. Fine. That's a chemistry you're looking at. And is it red, you have a redness there?		
728	C:	Well, it has a cedarish —		
729	P:	Cedarish color. There's some red in there, isn't there?		
730	C:	Yeah [Yes.].		
731	P:	Isn't that interesting? It's a cedar box.*	45:00	
732	C:	It's got black on it.		
733	P:	It's got black on it.		
734	C:	And I think there's still got the oil residue all over it.		
735	P:	Neat. We're getting a blend. The, the, the, the brain is beginning to blend this.*	45:15	
736	C:	Yeah [tentative "Yes."].		

737	P:	[You see???], it's[???] fragments. [When???] The brain doesn't know, it'll scatter, and it will divide the problem into parts. And we have to just hang out and watch the parts come together. If, that, don't quite make sense [???].		737-740. Levine's big-bang scatter theory reiterated.
738	C:	*Well, we're getting, it's becoming more, it's a cedar box permeated.	45:30	738-739. The surface of oil is now entering into the frozen natural energy characterized by the cedar box, now loosening up the wooden characteristic of the box.
739	P:	Um-hum [OK.].		
740	C:	Instead of encompassed, it's now permeated by oil.		
741	P:	Fantastic. Isn't that interesting how that works?*		
742	C:	Yeah [Yes.]. The box just got [is a lot???] bigger.* It's turning. I keep getting this image of when it opens, what's in it is a park * or a, like Yellowstone or something like that.	46:00	
743	P:	U'mum [OK.], umhum [OK.].		
744	C:	And a bear. A big black bear.		A bear appears—and later the woods (woulds?) the puns brain offers tempt us into narrative).
745	P:	All right. Wow!		
746	C:	And I know that the bear is my, um, * I don't know what you'd call him, but the....	46:15	A sacred healing energy is identified.

TRAUMA ENERGETICS

A SESSION

747	P:	Beast?
748	C:	Yeah, that [but???] connect with the,
749	P:	Medicine
750	C:	my
751	P:	medicine animal.
752	C:	animal, yeah. *	46:30
753	P:	Friend?
754	C:	The black bear is my companion.
755	P:	Yep [OK.].
756	C:	And obviously is a protector.
757	P:	Yep [Yes.].
758	C:	And the black bear is kind of walking away.
759	P:	Yeah [Yes.].
760	C:	Walking, but wanting me to follow and looking back.
761	P:	Um-hum [OK.].
762	C:	And we're going into the woods.
763	P:	Um-hum [OK.].

764	C:	The bear's oily.*	46:45	
765	P:	Um-hum [OK.].		
766	C:	The bear is real sad.* We're just going deeper into the woods. He's slowing down. Real sad.	47:00	
767	P:	Um-hunh [OK.].* Stay in the narrative, just for a while. It's ok to do that, er, don't you think?	47:15	I identify the narrative, but think it is interesting to hang out there for a while to see what happens. The energetics of the situation are complex but organic, infused with whatever the life force is, into animal form.
768	C:	Uh-huh [Yes.].		
769	P:	Just to see. Then if we get stuck, we'll go back * into the energetic.	47:30	
770	C:	The trees, the trees are so, the trees represent, the trees represent, there's nothing but* just these pegs	47:45	
771	P:	Uhm-hm [OK.].		
772	C:	of bark coming up. You can't see any green. There's no green on the ground.		
773	P:	Un-hunh [OK.].		

#	Sp.	Text	Time	Commentary
774	C:	But maybe everything is muddy. But not, *but brown, not muddy black,	48:00	774-775. Brown may express energetic bruise, but not held energy. In some ways we are, as it were, on the downhill side of this exploration, because brown can be resolved relatively quickly because it is a color (active) vibration, thus implying some healing potential within its bruised or wounded status. Trauma black also can be dissolved, yet its inapproachable facade or surface evokes ambivalent vectors. The pre-arrival homecoming sequences of the *Odyssey* express this ambivalence.
775	P:	Umum [OK.].*	48:15	
776	C:	just the bear.		
777	P:	Um-hum [OK.].		
778	C:	under this tree,		
779	P:	Um-hum [OK.].		
780	C:	It's like we're having, we're making our way through all of these *obstacles, that's* caging[???].	48:45	
781	P:	Uhmhm [OK.]		
782	C:	I, I don't get it.		
783	P:	Uhmhm [OK.].		
784	C:	This....		

785	P:	The energy is what for each of them? Drop into the energetic, see what it, it, is it, there a color to it?		We drop into the energetic, and I announce it as such, not keeping the technique hidden. I do that even more now than when this was recorded.
786	C:	Brown.		
787	P:	It's brown. The, the trees are brown.		I intuit spine and meningeal trauma, possibly damage [see 788-791] all of which I intuit can be resolved (healed?) at this level.
788	C:	Uh-huh [Yes.].		
789	P:	The stumps?		
790	C:	Yeah [Yes.]. I keep going up though, but I can't see the blue-green, any life to 'em.		
791	P:	Right. So how about going toward the..... Go into, go into the brown of the trees. Which, which interests you? Which, which, let's go into the energetic here. Brain* is having difficulty. And we can hang out at that level and think we're getting somewhere. But if we get the pattern to change, we've got to go into the energetic.	49:00	791-819. We strategize until there is a resolution. The energetic is showing a polarity here which becomes increasingly interesting as the client hovers in the complexity of trees and bear. What I find is that focusing energetically, the problematic areas are surprisingly located not at the gross surfaces, but at the right angle turns, or the places where facets join, or where there are two competing colors. These seem to be natural joinings, but their vector differences usually imply some supervalent forces holding the sides together at, say, right angles. Along the joining or abutting line is in fact a huge space which if focused on, may release significant information and change.

792	C:	Yeah [Yes (vaguely).].	
793	P:	So let's figure out. Shall we go into, you have into,* into the black coating, black, of the bear? We could go into [it], 'cause that has oil and that's some sign of some	49:15
794	C:	Yeah [OK.].	
795	P:	continued continuity.	
796	C:	Yeah [Yes.]. Yeah, let's do that.	
797	P:	Or we could go into the trees, the brown of the trees?	
798	C:	No, the trees are a distraction. * The trees are a constant something coming through.	49:30
799	P:	Hmm.	
800	C:	Now, the bear has sat down and is just looking.*	49:45
801	P:	OK, so we've got two colorations here.	
802	C:	Yeah [Yes.].	
803	P:	We've got a transition here between brown and, from between black and brown, which is	
804	C:	Right.	
805	P:	The brown, what you[we???]'ve been seeing that all along here .	50:00

806	C:	Yeah		
807	P:	in different forms, haven't we?*		
808	C:	Yeah [Yes.].		
809	P:	Right?		
810	C:	Yeah [Yes.].		
811	P:	So let's go back and forth. I want you to see if you can go into the black, as pure color, go into the black there.		811-812. We try to isolate the sensate experience of the contrast, to find just how exhausting it is for brain. What conscious thought, or what you and I would take as just ordinary camera panning, in fact contains often extreme vectors of stress. These may not be observed or sensated as distinctly in ideas or emotions as they may energetically in the colors.
812	C:	Well, *it's like I can go in, but it's a friendly black.	50:15	Here, the black may be functioning as a refuge, by protecting against entry into a very difficult place. There is a reversal of vector at this point, perhaps a clarification.
813	P:	Um-hum [OK.].		
814	C:	It's a, but then I find myself back out. It's like I*	50:30	Another reversal of vector.
815	P:	Um-hum [Yes.].		

816	C:	I, that, I can go in and then I have to…. OK, now, it's like being inside a porcupine.		The bear fur turns into a sharpness which brain identifies now as porcupine. We take up the parts and go into the color, a classic strategy.
817	P:	Yep [Yes.]. It's got quills?*	50:45	
818	C:	Yeah, and, and oil and quills.		
819	P:	Yep [Yes.].		
820	C:	Yep [Yes.].		
821	P:	Is there white on the quills?		
822	C:	White.		
823	P:	There's white.*	51:00	
824	C:	There's white dripping off the quills.		
825	P:	Whose pattern is this?*	51:15	825. I think I am premature here—maybe not.
826	C:	*Something I have to, I keep going through it.	51:30	Her response is describing the pattern .
827	P:	Um-hum [OK.]. Yep, I think that's a good answer.* I'll ask it again and see what, see what it, brain offers. Whose pattern is this?	51:45	From here on in there appears s real completion where there had been none. The bear—animal spirit—leads us. We follow the directions on the package (nature). The levels of integration now are at such a subtle and direct level and with a speed and comprehensiveness that it is impossible to imagine verbal rendering as being anything comparable to what is being observed and noted here.

828	C:	There's something very native Indian.		
829	P:	Yeah [Yes]. * Um-hum [OK.].*	52:00 52:15	
830	C:	It's like there's immanent[???]. It's time to* clear on. And as I said that, all this, I've got this picture of this huge sky, and vastness, and white, * white, white.	52:45	
831	P:	White stuff		
832	C:	White. No, not white. Not white. Air. See through.		My intuition is that this is a higher level of resolution than color, including white, which still expresses some incarnate holding of personality.
833	P:	Um-hum, yes, yes, that's the way. Stay with that, [???] [What happens as???] the chemistry resolves?		
834	C:	Um,* relief.	53:00	
835	P:	Yeah [Yes.].		
836	C:	Um, it's like the world opens.		
837	P:	Yup.		
838	C:	The green, the trees, and nature, and then that coloring.		
839	P:	Wow. There's green on the trees?*	53:15	

TRAUMA ENERGETICS

259

A SESSION

840	C:	Yeah [Yes.].		
841	P:	That's a real transformation.		
842	C:	Yeah [Yes,], it really feels like it. It's like moving through the light. And then the, finally getting through it. And these, the* clean[ness???] of air.	53:30	
843	P:	Umhum [OK.].		
844	C:	The bear is over here smiling, now.		
845	P:	(Laughter.)		
846	C:	(Laughter.) He's the nicest bear. This is just the most wonderful friend.*	53:45	
847	P:	I'm moved by that.		
848	C:	It's real-, me, too.		
849	P:	something[???]		
850	C:	It is real good. It's like what I've left is, you know, *by turning [my???] back, what's behind me is the swimming pool and Mom and Dad's fighting and anger and being a child and feeling like I had to* take that on or stand up to [th]em.*	53:30 53:45 54:00	850-873. There is some new "turning away" or distancing, and the insight [line 850] is OK but not where the movement is. Brain recapitulates the movement to orient itself *vis-à-vis* the new information.
851	P:	Um-hum [Yes.].		

852	C:	And I was the one in the family that always. It was like Mom, or [Nice???, or Varry???—members of the family], or anybody could stand up to all of it, so I would.		
853	P:	Yep [OK.].	54:15	
854	C:	With this fear. And I created something, *like a protector, to help me do it.		
855	P:	Right.		
856	C:	And maybe that's part of what the bear represents for me		
857	P:	Um-hum [OK.].		
858	C:	is that. And that's, that's kind of behind, and just moving* like towards the, just slowly moving past, or moving. [And], like, it let me turn around and look, and then it just started to sliding backwards.		858-859. Critical to this approach is the spatial rendering of the chemistry.
859	P:	So it's moving into some past?*	54:30	I am watching with her, trying to make sense of behind, past, etc.
860	C:	Yeah [Yes.].		
861	P:	Um-hum [OK.]. It's moving out of a tunnel.		We are coming into a new sequence.

#	Speaker		Time	
862	P:	Yep [Yes.]. I think that's the history, you know, that's the history "section" of the brain, is, is reorganizing that.		I offer an orientation, perhaps a bit hokey, but not so bad when our focus is on the energy and our attempt to connect words to the energy. Then even casual suggestions or strategies are just that. They may be withdrawn, midstream, as it were, or renegotiated. It appears the primacy of the energetic which keeps the statements "honest," not their truth. Many therapists insist on certain interpretations, sometimes driving clients to the wall. Here, no verbal overlay is sacred, or written in stone.
863	C:	Yeah [OK.].*	54:45	
864	P:	Without [???] fear, too much trouble.		
865	C:	Yeah [Yes.], that's what I feel. Boy, brain is really cool.		865-870. Her appreciation of her own process is real.
866	P:	Isn't it, something? (Laughter.)*	55:00	
867	C:	It's really cool.		
868	P:	Is this fun?		
869	C:	This is really neat.		
870	P:	Yeah [Yes.], you're doing beautifully with it. Controlling [???] following it.		
871	C:	There's a real sense of a, of* a clean.	55:15	

872	P:	Um-hum [Yes.]. Throughout the cells, th[e], ha[s], at the cellular level maybe?	872-873. **I encourage clients to sense themselves as cellular as well as more densely structural and organ-dominated. When the stress patterns depart, it is because they depart throughout a holding pattern in the entire body—archipelagoes of cells similarly torqued in perhaps the same quadrant of the cell (upper left hand corner, to offer a simplistic example). When the patterns are allowed to complete, other processes, too deep for human understanding, may rework. The only problem is getting used to this kind of witnessing and transformation. It requires a tolerance for the chemistry as primary, the interest in witnessing change at this level, and the ability to increasingly respect our capacity for going not exactly toward the pain, though that has some initial efficacy as a strategy. Rather, the client focuses specifically on the black (as color, or to put it more accurately, as absence of vibration), which involves the renegotiation of our interface with the held-energy system and its current domination of whole sections of our mindbody system. As so-called personalities, we are like pinballs bumping up against posts of held-energy which we mistakenly read as solid. No wonder these self-knowledges we tragically develop primarily in response to held-energy systems are as houses built on sand.
873	C:	Yeah [Yes.]. Yeah. I got a lot of oil out.	Some would say she is speaking metaphorically. I think what she is speaking about is a traumatic pattern now "dissolved" or completed, a stress pattern resolved.

#	Speaker	Utterance	Time	Commentary
874	P:	Yep [Yes.]. Have you got all of it out?*	55:30	At times I check to see if the pattern is gone. If the client feels it has merely moved to the side, or has whizzed off-stage, then I think it will return. Time of course, will tell. When the pattern goes through the permutations as it has done, here, I feel more secure about pattern recurrence. The bottom line is if it recurs, we haven't gotten to the bottom of the pattern yet. That is the most efficacious strategy I know to take, and it can change our orientation toward chronic pain, for example. The movement from the stress-free chemistry back into the pattern has to be strategized so that we do not become discouraged.
875	C:	Hunh, at this moment I don't feel it		
876	P:	Fantastic. So		876-905. We try to accurately describe the limits and extent of our success.
877	C:	or see it.		
878	P:	in this place,		
879	C:	Yeah [Yes.].		
880	P:	in this place we've got it out.		
881	C:	Yeah [Yes.].		
882	P:	If it comes back, we'll, in another place, we'll get it out.		
883	C:	It has to be in another place, because this place,* that, that all that black is gone. I mean	55:45	
884	P:	Watch the chemistry of that. That's a, it...		

885	C:	it's gone in file[d???].	
886	P:	There you go.	
887	C:	It's gone and it's moved back behind me.* And then it's like, just moved off to different little boxes.	56:00
888	P:	Yeah [OK]. Places you can refer to if you need to know what's there.	
889	C:	Yeah [Yes,], but they're not black.	
890	P:	They're not black. So we've changed that chemistry.*	56:15
891	C:	Yeah [Yes.]. I mean it's like Mom and Dad were put on a shelf. And the boat is on a shelf.	
892	P:	That sounds pretty good.	
893	C:	And even the little space ship, M&M* whatever (laughter).	56:30
894	P:	The M&M spa-, (laughter) the M&M. Eh- th', the space ship M&M.	
895	C:	doesn't even have a black center. It has, I don't know,* [???]* some kind of take [???]integ.... It has a, a depth to it, but it doesn't have black.	56:45 57:00
896	P:	Yeah [Yes.].	

A SESSION

897	C:	That's on the shelf over here. (Laughter.)	
898	P:	That's on the shelf too. So the brain is now,* I think that's a, d[oes] that feel like a good sort of completion	57:15
899	C:	Oh, yeah [yes,],	
900	P:	place?	
901	C:	it's just a wonderful place.	
902	P:	I now [??? ear]. Now we can talk about what, what to do, you know, besides drink some water.	
903	C:	Yeah [Yes.].* 'Cau[se] I love black.	57:30
			Black appears to have at least two vector functions: both are to protect, but at different levels of immersion into the held-energy system. Clients find that they enter some black because it senses as safe in that it in effect conveys, "You can't go any further into the dangerous chemistry I conceal." The other function is decidedly ambivalent: to ward off and conceal, countered by a demand to attend because it is an energetic blip, a traffic bump, but one which cannot be recognized or penetrated or solved. Here I think the client expresses brain's confidence that it can approach the black, at least in this place. And maybe others.
904	P:	Things peeling out.	
905	C:	Rain drops on out, yeah.	
906	P:	[Laughter.]	

907	C:	It's almost like what it feels like is happening, all the black drops are just moving down.		907-918. The chemistry seems to be reworking here. There are a series of playful comments—the process is joked about, simplified, etc. Playful as it was meant to be, I don't like line 914 and didn't, even as I said it. It felt outside the process and reflects some holding place (ego) in me. When I continue to make errors now, clients develop a sensitivity to such boundary compromises, and it becomes a function of our relationship that we are mutually, playfully vigilant.
908	P:	Yep [Yes.]. Yep [Yes.].*	57:45	
909	C:	It must be coffee. (Laughter.)		
910	P:	Right. (Laughter.) You've been drinking too much coffee, and that's the whole answer to your problem. (Laughter.)		
911	C:	(Laughter.) That's the whole problem. (Laughter.)		
912	P:	(Laughter.) Isn't that funny? I love it.*	58:00	
913	C:	No, the coffee's not quite dark enough.		
914	P:	Right. (Laughter.) I'll put a little cream in it.		
915	C:	No, that did feel just great.		

916	P:	Yeah [Yes.] Good. Well, we got, we got through something.* It, it had a magnitude about it.	58:15	916ff. I indicate some parameters of appreciation for what has been accomplished. In the winding down phase, before we separate our energy fields, and especially afterwards, there is chatting and commentary about the directions the session took, further possibilities for work, possible responses to look out for, etc.
917	C:	Un-hunh [Oh, yes.].		
918	P:	I think for looking at something I thought you might have suggested when you started, you know, something there for us.*	58:30	
919	C:	Well, I think so too.		
920	P:	So it was a good job [show???].		
921	C:	Yeah [Yes.].		
922	P:	OK, so we're, it's wonderful. It's, um, I do feel the completion.		
923	C:	Uh-huh [Yes.].		

			Time	Commentary
924	P:	I sense that, * and I, so that sort of feels OK to leave. But I must tell you this. You know, the fundamental energy is quite/in fact [???] unbelievable. I've just had a wonderful time.	58:45	924-926. ** I reflect on my enjoyment experiencing connection at this level. Some of this commentary comes from trying to eliminate the retraumatizing factors encompassed in the idea of transference. In this strategy, where the energetic has been met, but not intruded upon, and the separation well negotiated, then the residue of trans-ferential process may be minimized. Transference occurs, I believe, when there is a denial of the energetic and an unwillingness to provide direct physical connection, negotiated as above. My appreciation is direct and personal, and states some sense not of insufficiency, but of sufficiency. Where I do not feel that, I renegotiate the energetic with the client by discussing the limits of boundary delineations.
925	C:	That's really good.		
926	P:	So,		
927	C:	Good/Love[???] connecting.		
928	P:	So you can understand the difficulty* in separating.*	59:00 59:15	
929	C:	Yeah [Yes.].		

#	Speaker		Time	Commentary
930	P:	So I, I'd like some advice, again. What does primitive brain say is the way that we're gonna, our bodies going to separate? We're bonded on other levels.		930-931. The problem becomes direct and physical, literal. The client now describes what needs to happen on the move-ment level, after a prolonged contact with my hands under the client's head. We are partners in the process, with the client taking the initiatory lead, and I check that out intuitively to see if I can follow what the client indicates.
931	C:	Well, this time* it's almost, yeah, this time it's almost that the.... Instead of going out this time, it's almost like it needs to come [indicates with gesture]....	59:30	931-933. Here the client indicates that unlike during a former session, where she directed my hands to go to the side of her head, here she says they should go up the back of her neck to the top of her head.
932	P:	Come up.		
933	C:	Uh-huh [Yes.].		
934	P:	All right. Let's do that. Can you tell me if it needs to change, or if I am not doing it* the best way? Can you go back? There we go, uh, we can use a little Rolfing, uh, roll here. * Going to [dis]connect [from???] your hair, but I'm going to moon shop[???stop]. Is that OK?	59:45 60:00	Referring to some Rolfing pressure and turning with Rolfing intention, something I don't do, except here the client, a Rolfer, was very familiar with Rolfing. I was experimenting with her to show some relationship between what we had been doing and what she might be doing with her Rolfing.
935	C:	Yeah [Yes,], it's great.		
936	P:	'Cause there's a lot of very interesting pressure there which, and I think you should just hold, let, let have happen and not [rush???].		

		++ *End of Side One, Tape One* ++ ++ *Beginning of Side Two, Tape One* ++	++For purposes of general convenience and accuracy, I have adjusted the transfer time from one side of the tape to the other by rounding it off to the next minute, though the actual time was about twenty seconds. A couple of spoken lines were thus not recorded, and not included here.
937	C:	* ...you're taking with you, 'cause I sure feels good, a s[ense?], a whole bunch of that, um....	61:00 — Here the client indicates that I am "taking with" me some of the toxicities which she has been dealing with. This presents an issue of boundaries, some of which are "real," some of which require a talking through. If I take on the toxicities and those are not adequately described or circumscribed, the energetic becomes an arena for projection and transference, not of resolution. There will be more work to do with her on this issue in a later session. Because of the length of the session already, I make a decision not to bring more into the lesson than our traffic can bear.
938	P:	Um-hum [Yes,], that crud.	
939	C:	Yes, * it's leaving. As, as you move, it's moving on out of my, um, being, my, my [energy, auric] 'sfield [???field. steel.]	61:15
940	P:	Your density,	
941	C:	Yeah [Yes.].	
942	P:	Yes, exactly. Well, * that's one of the reasons why we have to do this sequentially, so that I don't, I don't take it on.	61:30

#	Speaker	Text	Time
943	C:	Right.	
944	P:	But that it leaves.	
945	C:	But it's almost like, yeah, it's like it's leaving. The client experiences the toxicity being taken out as I move my hands away. That is not my intention; I am not sure that can be done except after some greater examination between us about boundaries and energy. My focus is non-intentional, non-transference-inducing. It is energetically sufficient, and non-invasive, hence under those conditions of sufficiency without violation, brain will offer up the trauma for resolution.	
946	P:	Let's see if we can negotiate that. Let's play with that. I am concerned that the boundaries between us stay firm and appropriate as we take leave, in order that both of us not be retraumatized. We are at equal risk in this matter. We need to align around the issue of how I get rid of the pattern as well as she in this. I believe I am a model for taking responsibility in a way which most clients have not experienced. Energetically, clients withhold to protect the other person (parent, therapist, lover, whatever), and so continue to take on the sins, as it were, to retraumatize over the core energetic patterning. It is important to remember that these patterns do not yield to pressure or violence, even though they get neurochemically laid in by violence or abuse; and that their conclusion is in some kind of self-dissolution.	
947	C:	Yeah.	61:45
948	P:	*Make sure that that's.... 'cause you won't feel so good if you think you're just dumping it.	

#	Speaker	Text	Time	Notes
949	C:	No, it's like it's in your.... It's like you're just scraping it off.		949–951. We renegotiate—the client is telling me how it is.
950	P:	That's fantastic.		
951	C:	And then it'll....		
952	P:	And then it will come off.		
953	C:	Yeah [Yes.].		
954	P:	Watch that happen. * There, that [energy] turns it out, your forehead is now free [inaudible???], when you stay in that energy.	62:00	
955	C:	Yeah [OK.].*	62:15	
956	P:	Just a little. Now, I'm about two inches away, [???inaudible] at the crown of your head.		956–957. Usually the client has her eyes closed, or is concentrating on something else, so that I keep her posted on what exactly my hands are doing.
957	C:	Uh-huh [OK.].		
958	P:	Now I'm coming [a bit???]* around. I'm just going to spread it out sort of like a big headdress here	62:30	
959	C:	Umm.		
960	P:	so that....		

TRAUMA ENERGETICS

A SESSION

#	Speaker	Dialogue	Time	Commentary
961	C:	Um, the black is dripping off.*	62:45	The black is dripping off (her "inner" screen), but it is not disappearing. Hence my framing commentary that there may be more ahead for brain to experience here. It is like allowing for homework.
962	P:	Good. Now that's a piece of the puzzle that you haven't known how to do, right?		962-972. The application of these strategies hopefully gives the client a sense of freedom in an otherwise constricted configuration.
963	C:	Yeah [Yes.]. How you get rid of the black?		
964	P:	Yep [Yes.].		
965	C:	Yeah [Yes.].*	63:00	
966	P:	Now my, my understanding is in terms of strategy will be, there may be a point where you may get the pattern coming back in another shape. And you'll,		
967	C:	Un-hunh [Yes.].		
968	P:	you'll want to go into the molecule,* in whatever shows up in black, you'll want to go into the black in another, in an additional way.	63:15	

969	C:	Um-hum [OK.]		
970	P:	In other words, this is a very important piece of information that we've gotten brain to understand; that it can get rid of the black.		
971	C:	Un-hunh [Yes.].*	63:30	
972	P:	And maybe that will be enough. But in terms of your preoccupation with say somebody like [a person client had mentioned previously] who zaps you with		972-973. Indicating someone else who the client feels attempts to energetically control her.

973 | C: | Unhunh [Yes.].

973-980.** I skirt advice, though now would state more about that area where advice is offered. Advice is inappropriate to this kind of work if we remain watchful of the energy. The intrusiveness of intentionality is challenged here because the brain chemistry does not appear to change except when we unlock it in its own order. There may be some intention in the decision to look and to witness, but that is usually inspired by pain or discomfort, at an inner or even physically manifest level. Most intentionality may be determined by those factors, but that isn't what most people think about when they talk about intentionality. Who would say, "I am motivated to intend by my pain."? I think most decisions are made in response to our held-energy systems. Clients and I find choice experienced from a position of *resolved* trauma scary beyond ordinary imagination, ye t I think that is what we know we must experience, in order to see the Godhead, reality, our essential nature, whatever. Are not the structures which curb this expansiveness cultural, genetic, and psychodynamic, all having retraumatizing potentiality?

When someone says, "Well, are you going to give up all civilization, all patternings? Some patternings are good, etc. The vision you share is too ethereal, too spiritual, too classically utopian," my response is to suggest that this may be the state of the art, the place to which this journey leads. There are lots of precedents toward this kind of clarity in the history of current humanity, and their implication and implementations have been only partial. Those who challenge us to be clear are usually destroyed in the victim and abusehood which such clarity unlocks. (Continued next cell).

		63:45	(*Continued from above cell*). abusehood which such clarity unlocks. If we cannot experience clarity, then what are we able to do? I ink we perpetrate, in the name of morality, and exigency. The movement filtered through public morality forms and customs is retraumatizing and perpetrative. All declarations about morality lead up to the door of the energetic, and have to be dropped there, as they have had to be throughout recorded history, both in the history of ideas and the history of movement. I intuit all narratives must dissolve at the same doorstep in order for us to experience the frightening freedom which we say we want so badly. Intentionality takes us to the interface between the energetic and its incarnation (its blending, its manifestation) in the mindbody, in its structure and in the overt as well as the covert movements it manifests (does and is).
974	P:		by pulling on these patterns, you know, pulling for resolutions, patterns come up *in your [system, psyche???]. You don't know how he's doing it, you know. This may, this may help you.
975	C:		Yeah [Yes,], when I[???] let it drop off.	That is her solution, not mine. I bring an issue which she is concerned about in the narrative [she mentioned it in conversation some time before the session] into juxtaposition with the energetic in an informational context.
976	P:		Let it drop off.	I stay next to her.

977	C:	I have this, this sense right now almost being, *uh, connected with, uh, my, um, with the bear. Just, just this by encompassing me, * um, a [???] connection. But more so than I think I've ever even known. I've always had him as a traveling companion. * It's really neat.	64:00 64:15 64:30	977-981. I view this again as a neurochemistry, some sort of completing companionate integrative process, though in its animal form, it may be still taking narrative form. I feel its developmental appropriateness, though unlike a teddy bear, the process encompasses a profoundly adult integration of intuition and need. I would be happy as she in a similar chemistry.
978	P:	Yep [Yes.].		
979	C:	[???]to stand by him[???] I have with him[???inaudible]		

| 980 | P: | Yep [Yes.], yeah. Now, it may be that the, that if, if you get, if you find it coming, coming back, and, you know, the brain is cycling through again and wants something else from that information.* | 65:00 | 980-1006. Because the energy, coded black, is now in a living animal form, I believe we are much closer to the core traumatic pattern, as contrasted to when it was in the oil shape. And the image tells us that we are on the right track, that there is an escorting process; we have established a working rather than hostile, frightened or come-here/go-away relationship to the black. This reunion, if you will, is happily experienced, in its more appropriate and natural enfleshed form. However, I am still pursuing the black, because I know it will come forward again, perhaps even very soon, given the satisfying chemical "platform" which the client has just achieved. Brain has a direction, and it will be able to follow the sequence of information it has taken in more than it did before this session. I am structuring the anticipated next phase of the work, so that she will not be totally surprised, or if something comes up, we may learn more about the trauma mechanism by referring to this comment. One of the major disappointments clients experience with this work is the transition out of the initial high which occurs. One client said, "I think I screwed it up," when the pattern returned a few days later." In some patterns, it has taken me a very long time to welcome the next phase of black as an achievement, rather than a setback. It appears the fulcrum of that transition is critical for brain to get interested in, and to learn from. (*Continued next cell*). |

#				
981	C:	Un-huh [OK.].		(*Continued from above cell*). For me, narrative and expressive approaches tend to confound that shift. I believe clients can be educated toward this anticipation, though the evidence of the Christian Church's experience with explaining the parallel relationship between, say, the held-energy system of Good Friday and the movement of Easter suggests that in the midst of the experience of so-called trauma completion, no one finds it easy. Yet it is within that mechanism that the important, transforming information to be valued by the brain is contained, even though the specifics of it may be invisible.
982	P:	you may find yourself in some ways reengaging with black at another level.		
983	C:	Uh-huh [OK.].		
984	P:	And you may find that there's more for you to know.		
985	C:	Un-huh [OK.].*	65:15	
986	P:	But you've gotten a major piece of it out today. And maybe all of it.		986-987. Summary statements—appreciations of the session. I am still making comments of acknowledgement, strategy, whatever, after a session. I don't know whether to comment or not, but sometimes some reentry into the verbal centers of ordinary thinking are useful. The relational aspects of the commentary—we are equals here in facing the energy—both experimental and equals in perspective, need some talking through.
987	C:	Uh-huh [OK.].		987-988, 1004-1005. More consolidation of how to appreciate the lesson. She has an understanding of this already.

#	Speaker	Text	Time
988	P:	I can't tell.	
989	C:	Well, yeah.	
990	P:	So we really did	
991	C:	It's great.	
992	P:	we did a lot. * And brain will have to hover through it, in and out of this process.	65:30
993	C:	Oh, yeah [OK].	
994	P:	And you'll go back and forth and sort of, but don't, you know, if you, if you.... And the more you get the green and the clear, the more whatever residue * of further traumatic process	65:45
995	C:	Keeps	
996	P:	will come forward, and you should anticipate it. And when you get the good stuff, you realize you're, you know, you're "setting a table before them, before me, before me," you know, "in the presence of mine enemies," * you know, that old	66:00
997	C:	Oh, yeah.	
998	P:	psalm?	
999	C:	Um-hum [Yes.].*	66:15

TRAUMA ENERGETICS

1000	P:	So you just, and you welcome the enemies to the table and say, "I'm getting this ready for you guys."	
1001	C:	That's what the Pleidieans kept saying: "Welcome the dark."	
1002	P:	Yep [Yes.].*	66:30
1003	C:	And then [???] your educators and then	
1004	P:	Yeah [Yes.].	
1005	C:	changing[???].	
1006	P:	Yep [Yes.]. And that's what's your path.	
1007	C:	It's a constant class (laughter).	
1008	P:	Well, I don't think brain can usually process it alone, not	
1009	C:	I'm sure.	
1010	P:	in the critical traumatic places, 'cause	
1011	C:	Yeah [OK].	
1012	P:	the trauma message is *" Don't go in the door." "Cause it's, you know, it's black, and it's attractive and that's what comes up five times a second[s??? '(a)nd] to resolve, but "Don't go there." My current sources suggest about ten times per second.	66:45
1013	C:	Hmm.	
1014	P:	So you you're caught [going] back and forth.	

1015	C:	Uh-huh [OK.].	
1016	P:	And you'll ask, "What the hell am I supposed to do?" And you'll head back into narrative, *thinking, "Oh, well now, I haven't understood the situation."	67:00
1017	C:	Uh-huh [tentative].	
1018	P:	You get back into suffering, into the soap opera.	1018-1021. I try to indicate the nature of the strategy she has just accomplished. What may distinguish this approach is that it makes a sharp delineation between narrative and energy at the level of the color. This seems to be important in the delineation of what remains or what there is to do. Learning information at the vibrational level is quite different from at a narrative level. Elements of the former can be intuiteded from the latter, while elements of the narrative are less likely to be at the pure color level, though the issues which they present graphically are certainly narratable.
1019	C:	Uh-huh [Yes.]. Instead of [???]	
1020	P:	Instead of staying into the black. And you may not be able to do it just by yourself.	
1021	C:	Yeah [OK.].*	67:15

1022	P:	You may need someone, a person, to support you. Not to do anything; I wasn't doing anything today.		"Doing" here means not forcing or intending the result in traditional ways, by substituting ideas, thought patterns for the client. What I "do" is to try and follow the directions of the brain as to how to unlock the held-energy system so brain itself can understand it, not "me" nor the client's usual sense of self).
1023	C:	Staying in the black.		
1024	P:	Just find it. And it isn't something you can do *just by.... I mean you can sort of give guidance, but I think you, the brain has to get attracted to it.	67:30	We are not looking at volition here. We have to figure out how to lead a reluctant brain to the water, not to drink, but to focus.
1025	C:	Um-hum [Really?].		
1026	P:	As the substance		
1027	C:	Look at the black.		
1028	P:	That's what I really want to do. It's an acquired taste.* Follow it and watch what happens.	67:45	I share my own journey on this, particularly when it starts to smell of dogma, rather than strategy, from me or from the need of the client to have dogma. Here I think it was me.
1029	C:	Um-hum [OK.]. That's neat. Well, that was a wonderful session.		
1030	P:	Thank you.*	68:00	
1031	C:	No, thank you.		

| 1032 | P: | for doing that. Can you say the magic words, "I'm in my body and it's OK?" | ** Speaking of dogma, here is a strategy which I conclude each session with. After one session a client was upset because he did not feel grounded, and his therapist advised this phrase as a way of "grounding" after the work. I have always wondered about end-of-session body work where some of the effect is compromised by the last finishing touches. I have often felt irritated by perfectionists whose gestures seemed not to take into account the new sensations I was experiencing and wanted to explore. In some cases I have felt some moves made a difference, and in these cases, I always make some intuitive energetic moves as I separate, and then touch the sides of the legs and feet.

I sometimes keep contact with clients as they move into the vertical—we negotiate at every point, so that the energetic bonding is suitably respected. When I have taken my hands from the back of their neck (if that is the sequence we are following), I ask clients to get off the table into a vertical standing position any way they can. I encourage them to learn in the process, staying with the energy as a kind of developmental focus. One classical pianist slid headfirst off the side of the table, dragged himself underneath it and rolled out the other side, coming to a kneeling position at the other side. Clients will often walk around the room in various ways as a way of bringing themselves into "Boston" time. In short, I urge clients now to stay with the energy and not to reconnect with ordinary movement ordinarily, such as by stretching. Though not in this particular case, *(Continued next cell).* |

#	Sp		Time
1033	C:	" I'm in my body and it's OK." Real nice.	
		(Continued from cell above), this sometimes involves a rather extensive process, sometimes taking as long as 15 minutes. Our goal is not to retraumatize, but to enable both of us to disconnect with some modicum of energetic wholeness, so that transference does not occur (a sure sign of retraumatization from this perspective). When clients are doing this work by themselves lying in bed, for example, I think it important to sense how the energy infuses or guides the grosser density of physical movement rather than is dragged by it, or is in rebellion against the impacted, impaled energy of the held-energy system and becomes impulsive and dissociated, where most of us are.	
1034	P:	Good. OK, let's see how [you can???] go to the side of the table???].	
1035	C:	Um-hum [OK.] * I'm glad to. Hmm, I feel [in a] very clear place. Oh my...	68:15
1036	P:	Yep [OK.]..	
1037	C:	Hmm. Oh.	
1038	P:	Yep [OK.].	
1039	C:	Hmm. Cool. I'm pleased.	
1040	P:	*OK. Let me, um, just touch the sides of your legs	68:30
1041	C:	OK.	

1042	P:	and the bottoms and the tops of your feet just to be, so you don't, get some floor [grounding] so whatever. And I liked when, when you went, you were, I mean, there was a point when we were staying in the narrative and it felt grand to do that		1042-1061. Further commentary as she is getting oriented. Sometimes I am giving clients time to gather in their process, other times I think I intrude, either out of my own patterning or to cover the energetic separation. Some clients "get" a point in an important way in this after-session; for them, it is like taking an additional something away. Here also is a shared collegiality which demystifies our relationship, and with feedback, prepares for the integration of the information and the context of, if desired, the next session(s).
1043	C:	Hmmm-hmm [Yes.].		
1044	P:	and then when we got stuck we went, we went into the color,		
1045	C:	Hmm.		
1046	P:	into,* back into the energy, that's when the movement started [stopped???]	68:45	
1047	C:	Um-hum [Yes.]. Um-hum [Yes.].		
1048	P:	The brain needs to go sometimes horizontally through narrative, but should not confuse that with the vertical drop into the energetic.*	69:00	
1049	C:	Into th'?		
1050	P:	Into the black or into the color,		

1051	C:	Umhm [OK.].										
1052	P:	going into the brown. 'Cause when you do that, then the whole landscape changes.										
1053	C:	Yeah [OK.]. Then there's open and,										
1054	P:	Yeah [Yes.].										
1055	C:	and new. It's neat. Thank you.										
1056	P:	Thank you.*	69:15									
1057	C:	I really enjoyed it. [Laughter.]										
1058	P:	[Laughter.]										
1059	C:	Now let me										
1060	P:	Yup [Yes.].										
1061	C:	stand up.										
1062	P:	Is this [OK?] Yes.										
1063	C:	Cool.										

1064	P:	And, uh, drink some water.	Fresh pure water seems a great way to conclude. I often say, "Literally and symbolically drink the water to flush out whatever toxicity residues remain in the system which need flushing. And to facilitate the integration of new information." Some clients can playfully estimate how long it will take to do this. I ask them to call me within a relatively short time to report what they are experiencing; the times vary depending upon the session and the experience of the client. We strategize for the next sessions, some of which may take place a long time later. Brain often needs a long time to absorb and delineate the new information. To this end, I urge them not to analyze, and to watch the brain recombining and reworking (new, sometimes absurd insights will occur), and to let brain do its work.
1065	C:	Yeah [Yes,], I will.	
1066	P:	And pee it [toxins] out. Yeah, there it is.	+++

End of Side Two, Tape One

CHAPTER SEVEN: ENERGY, THE SPIRIT, AND RELIGION

Friends: The following chapters carry the aforementioned insights about trauma into the realm of spirituality and its often wayward handmaidens, religion and myth. For some, this transition may be too quick or abrupt, or irrelevant. As more than one reader has noted, this stuff is not for everybody. For others this section may clarify how the smoke passes up through the crown chakra.

Political Religion

Major ventures into the mechanism of trauma establish social and personal beachheads which tend to evoke new embodiments of the energetic, often characterized as releases, cultural shifts, revolutions, etc. They also bring additional traumata and retraumatization, in the formation of religious and political dogma and political religion.

By political religion, I mean those social agencies, including churches and their structures, which sustain and moderate the common weal in communities. We could also view similarly positioned governmental agency such as legislatures as religious politics. Where we have a so-called separation of church and state, both groupings in fact borrow or claim attention from the other realm, based as both are on the same objectives, a safe, satisfying life for their constituencies. Churches and states hold similar, overlapping functions, appealing to similar claims to value delineation, allegiance, and understanding.

As group experiences, both contrast with those of individual spirituality. Are not the primary means of these agencies toward social order and continuity usually lineaged through indoctrination and pressures to conform?

The spiritual objectives surrounding the individualistic "longings" for worship, enlightenment, and the ending of suffering as implemented within the so-called self are real and sometimes met. Yet at certain points in the interaction between individual and group, they appear only a minor part, perhaps "loss leader" might be a better term, of the traditional agenda of political and religious institutions. These institutions have demanded allegiance, even when truth would carry their parishioners beyond them. Why is this?

Insofar as suffering motivates civilization, so-called civilization may be based upon the two-stage movement within the trauma mechanism. When our energy is balanced and vibrationally tuned to a certain "pitch," up comes traumatic patterning for resolution. Often these patterns are the point of origin for societal and cultural artifacts, such as constitutions, dogma, and architecture. Potentially, all manifestations of the trust-trauma sequence can be dropped when the patterns can be seen and dissolved.

While the dissolution of history envisioned by Hegel and Marx may be a politicized projection of the psychological experience of what integrity implies, history rarely dissolves. Or if it does, we don't hear about it. Aside from Gandhi's or perhaps Malcolm X's, when was the last time we read a biography of a public leader where his/her individual enlightenment(s) occurred, or much rarer, was the declared main course? Nonetheless, religious, and for that matter, political lineages promise such a time and experience for their constituency (cf. Jerusalem, Nirvana, Heaven, Marxism, Blake, Rousseau, etc.).

In the history of the West, it is curious how major religious groups evolve an understanding of the trauma mechanism which promulgates an initial release of energy, hope, and insight. With few and momentary exceptions, the leaders and their followers then proceed to perpetrate a most disturbing residual trauma pattern, dropping, as it were, the second shoe. Or, as with my childhood

acquaintance, going only so far into the problem and then eating the
rest of the banana whole.

Genesis and Origins

While it may seem contrary to their collective and widespread
application, it now seems wisest to admit we do not know quite what
the first chapters of Genesis describe. We are still finding out. The
longer as a culture we hang out with the text, the more we discover
and elaborate. One strategy is that, roughly speaking, the book of
Genesis, as its title suggests, is about origin.

At least four kinds of beginnings may be described in Genesis:

1. the origin of the universe, the initiation of Creation;

2. the beginning of humankind;

3. the beginning of individual awareness in each one of us as
we "incarnate,"

4. the point of origin of awareness in the listener-reader of
Genesis, who by definition dwells in or with dissociative process.

1. The beginning of Creation takes us immediately into
paradox, for beginnings imply a time before. Aquinas and others
resolve this problem by identifying God as the Unmoved Prime Mover
or Uncaused First Cause. While weighted with conflict and issues, the
story presented in the first chapters of Genesis at least represents a
convenient decision to focus discussion at the narrative level, rather
than the explosive, linear-mind-confounding paradox contained in time
itself.

Genesis concludes or obviates the paradox by providing a
point of origin for Creation. Juxtapose the paradoxical alternative
next to most fundamentalists, and, clutching at as well as rebelling
against narrative, they appear to throw their hands up in rage or
despair, and, if sensible, return to silence—actually not such a bad idea
for all of us. Genesis declares a point of origin for Creation.

How to approach this latter problem has been skillfully
elaborated by Big Bang physicists and astronomers, as well as others

trying to master time. The more physics theory comes to rephrase the problem of origin, the more congruent it becomes with the linguistic, poetic intuitions of Genesis, which attempt to narrate in linear terms something which may be beyond the capacity of our contemporary brains as we currently exercise them.

This should not surprise us, for our brain's basic structure has not changed over the past perhaps 10,000s of years. If we have only a right hand, all our tools and accomplishments will be determined by that fact. So any inroads made into knowing about the origin of Creation will be elaborated by scientific strategies set within the framework of our current cognitive and imaginative limitations.

2. Likewise, the beginning of human beings as a developing anthropological presence has deepened our insight into what is left in the theological paw of Genesis after that particular evolutionary thorn has been removed, and we can thank Darwin for that. Difficult as this revision of what Genesis is about has been, we have discovered lots of evidence to support a linear development which was not readily observed or understood before the mid-nineteenth century. As special apes, we can see how our genetic codes have altered, revised, and are revisable—all interesting, and important.

3. I think even more significant, for Jews and Gentiles, the origin vision of Genesis describes with telling accuracy the developmental process of individual experience, from the point of view of the infant. Initially, we are each the barely differentiated Spirit of God moving over the face of the amniotic waters until, delivering and delivered from the mother's womb, we "declare" Light. In our infancy, we are God, namely that which is, creating our world, dividing it into parts, naming it, just as we are being created and named, and our experience is becoming particulate.

In our relationship to the first person in the world, called traditionally the Mother—in Genesis it is called Adam—we intuitively fashion a truthful understanding of

a. how we come about: we are animated (star)dust;

b. how we are born: out of a body—people come from people;

c. how we differentiate: we separate and name—and in naming, we narrate;

d. how we relate to others: as the second person in the world, as infants, male and female, we "decline," fall, from being God to becoming Adam. No, with mother present as the person we see, we are not the first person, we are the second—so we become Eve; and

e. how we generate through time.

In terms of what *muthos* actually determines our action and sense of being, the scientific strategies of evolution may carry us to alternate visions of origin, but I intuit they do not substitute, yet, the power of Genesis. If we had to choose which is the map most helpful to our experience, most likely we would choose Genesis, or some similar myth, for it describes our developmental sequence from within the perspective of the infant. How this perspective generated in Genesis was gained and preserved is uncertain, but I find it a blessing of creative intuition.

4. The fourth origin, the origin of awareness within the person listening to Genesis, is the most problematic to describe, but Genesis attacks it with gusto and a certain primitive accuracy, prepared as we are in a way from the beginning of the first chapter. If we listeners assume we are in narrative, and we look for where narrative starts, Genesis has a startling and initially disturbing strategy—something in our experience is capable of going wrong, and something has gone wrong. Within the origin of our awareness is the origin of our suffering.

As we listen to Genesis, we are in dissociation, and this is a fundamental, ever-present fact of our ordinary experience, transmitted from the first parents to succeeding generations of children. Within the movement of the early stages of our life, held-energy systems have already compromised our clarity, have already made it difficult for us to apprehend the Godhead, as if we were expelled from a Garden of Eden. From perhaps the very conception of each person's life, the impact of this neurochemical process becomes increasingly apparent.

Mastering this mechanism also becomes important, such that adults return to it repeatedly, pouring over the *muthos* described in, say, Genesis, to align their understanding. It is not without reason that Bible-affiliated people resist removing this point of focus, critically placed as it has been for over a short 5,000 years. In some radical way, we read the Bible because we are in dissociation, in narrative, in imbalanced incarnation. Within the energetic, we would need no external guidance nor insight. Then we would be closer to God in the way animals and plants are.

The *anagnōrisis* about the trauma mechanism results at least in establishing the skewed nature of all narrative, the intrusion of a catastrophic vision of history, of causality, of self and community. It also generates a direction to go in, namely completion and restoration of the pre-apple (pre-windshield, pre-trauma) Garden experience.

That this is the first order of business for us challenged apes requires that we acknowledge the way in which our held-energy systems can predetermine all that we blithely think is free in us, until they are lifted off, or we discover the way to watch them lift themselves off. The origin of narrative can be located at trauma's gate, and we return to the held energetic to unseal its form and resultant rigidities.

From this point of view, the expulsion from the Garden is narratively congruent with the difficulty of entering the black, traumatically-encoded held-energy system, once the pattern has set in. That our traumata are experienced early in life is figured in the eating of the apple, suggesting feeding, birth, and before that, the intrauterine communication and absorption of energetic patternings.

Our brain's attempt to regain its original relationality with its own process becomes confounded with issues of guilt, shame, stupidity, blame, as well as the later seven deadly sins—all verbal, emotional, and addictive elaborations. These superstitions surround the impossibility of our brain decoding its very own invisible system. In this sense, Original Sin, though accurate, may be seen as superstitious elaboration upon the failure of brain to penetrate the black, violating its own protective informational code, as it were.

Original Sin

I remember how as children, we found the doctrine of Original Sin so difficult because it implied our imperfection and the possibility of being blamed before we had done anything to deserve it. Baptism reminded us that even from the almost start, there is something wrong. But what is wrong?

Catholics may have taken one side of the coin, proposing we are wrong from the start, an intriguing narrative strategy, while Jews maintained infants are not bad from the start, but that choice of direction, toward good or toward bad, is possible. Though referring indirectly to its factual presence, neither strategy appears to directly serve the insight of the continuity of trauma energetic or its invisible transmission. Somehow, as victims, we are blamed. Or made responsible.

Nonetheless, while the superstitious elaborations upon this essentially karmic strategy are daunting, its healing trajectory is equally formidable. For if the Original Sin strategy implies a sewer-scraping, cleansing function, we want to be able to apply it not halfway into our journey, when shifting vector direction takes enormous energy, but from the place where the patterns start. Original Sin goes back to the "first error" or "first choice" by the "first persons," Eve, with Adam, and mythically identifies the starting point.

Our infantile projective identification with our parent(s) seems all encompassing, and the doctrine of Original Sin takes us to a place where it can be reworked, presumably as far back as we need to trace it. If there is an error committed in the Garden, what is it? Who is responsible? Pride of personhood is one usual answer, with its implied values of arrogance, egocentrism, narcissism, ignorance, rebellion, and disconnection. We are caught where we lose sight of the Power which creates us. God sets things straight by excluding Adam and Eve from the Garden's initial bliss and sets a flaming sword at the Gates to keep us from reentering what is precious, too dangerous, for us to experience.

What makes this commentary on origins so compelling is that it reveals not only developmental process, but it also identifies the neurochemistry of trauma. What is crucial to the imagery of the flaming sword is that it compresses the chaos and reentry heating up of trauma "renegotiation," again Levine's term, and provides a scenario of denial which all of us employ in dissociation experience: "What (wrong) did I do?"

We are drawn into a concern with the point of origin of the pattern of suffering which we are "left with," East of Eden. Our figleaves are signs of our suffering, easy signals to read by God's watchful eye. Why are we expelled from wholeness? Is it our fault? What do we have to do to get back into balance and connection?

Furthermore, in our desire to relocate at the higher vibration of Edenic wholeness and balance, like traumatic brain function itself, in Genesis the energetic experience of the trauma is omitted. Brain merely attaches a parallel narrative, "She gave me fruit of the tree, and I ate," which describes with lethal easefulness the openness with which trauma information is instantaneously delivered, absorbed, and laid in in held-energy systems, as well as the forbiddenness of entering the black. But, in Genesis, I think, we do not know the situation which actually incites the trauma mechanism and sets the held-energy system into immotion. The apple is not the bottom line.

This narrative of transgression becomes politically embellished with patriarchal authoritarianism: "Don't mess with Father God and what He forbids." Furthermore, our neurochemical code states that to reenter the trauma locus (To) is dangerous, which may no longer be the case. Our neurons may have developed, myelinated, and reconfigured since the first occasion, and we may now be able to sustain ecstasy with greater mastery.

That eating of the fruit of the tree of the knowledge of good and evil may be not so much an action, but rather a place of energetic immobility becomes acknowledged collectively only after millennia, and personally perhaps over decades. Its narrative form is an imitation of trauma energetics.

When the trust-trauma sequence begins to be experienced, and, in part by its overlapping structure, Genesis reports this happens very early on, it seems we revert to narrative, rather than remain in the energy. Only self-realized individuals appear able to focus upon the energetic with significant, sustained consistency.

The serpent tempts us into narrative or activity, poised in rebellion from or denial of the black connundra, which are what really trouble us. As spine in trauma, or "blocked" kundalini, the serpent diverts us away from the energetic onto a detoured "path," or non-righteous formulation of self and activity.

From the position of dissociation, outside the held-energy system, the path of righteousness is viewed as straight and narrow. From within, the path is open and expansive, to the point of being boundless. We do not confuse the black of held-energy with the black of void. In dissociation, we eat the fruit of the tree of knowledge of good and evil and fall into the illusion of narrative causality. The life force is filtered through a prior traumatic grid. And we spend lifetimes in the backwaters of suffering, unable to release ourselves from the immobilities we subsequently engender.

Evil and the Trauma Mechanism

Are we bad for having this mechanism at work within us? Some preachers exhort us with the vision that we are, and that the only way out of the mechanism is to reform our vision of self and its covenant with God. The personal vision of this covenant promulgated by the Christian lineage has been characterized by diving into an awareness of the perpetrative patterning and its encrustations by naming it evil. This patterning is then personified, as intuition suggests, in the gestalt form of Satan. What better way to show where and how the pattern resides than to illustrate its humanoid resemblance and incarnate manifestation.

But evil appears to have a narrative, causal vector, so it is not surprising when we cannot come into the resolution of the evil pattern, even though we think we know it has a beginning. Evil, in

Satanic form or otherwise, can be, like "laziness," "stupidity," and "boredom," superstitious imagery which keeps us at a secondary, not primary energetic level of awareness. This is not to say that we cannot find "evil" in the world, or people living out this vibrational conundrum and doing great harm, but to characterize it as evil invites a perpetrative mirroring response, with very little real change in our inner experience of our own power.

Those who have come into the revisionary chemistry of conversion may express the resultant compassion either universally, or like St. Paul, carry out the process only partially. They continue to perpetrate, but at a different level. Many people appreciate St. Paul for that reason, not because he appears fully self-realized, but because he reflects the partial understanding which seems to be within most of our grasps. A greater integrity in this context is perceived, perhaps realistically, perhaps charitably, as inhuman. At its worst, such "settling for less" in the name of Paul may reduce the political and personal healing power of its advocates.

The Savior

In this century of abuse, the lineage of abuse continues to march forward for resolution at the political as well as at the most intimate personal levels, as individuals face the difficulty of finding the point of origin for the patterns which destroy them. If we look for a beginning for the source of our suffering in narrative, won't we then look for its ending in narrative as well? We shall embody that ending in the narrative form of a *savior* who brings us salvation. Like the Devil, the Savior is a point of focus in humanoid, gestalt form, and the Savior's struggles with the Satan or its ilk can provide a representation of the energetic hiatus from which brain reverts to narrative.

But I find the struggle between Satan and Savior is illusory and not holistically true, not at the energetically clear, non-traumatized level of experience. The source for our suffering may lie within historical memory, but its beginning lies outside of time, in traumatic patterning, itself an initially life-sustaining distortion.

We could easily misunderstand this position by pointing to, say, World War II or the American Civil War experiences, where the gestalt of the struggles appeared to take particularly distinct forms. Were there not recognizable evils vanquished? And the results of those struggles are clear enough. People died about the struggles, or thought they did. And people were saved, and not saved, from destructions.

Confronted by the interface between personal historical memory and traumatic patterning, who will deny that victims often perpetrate their trauma by staying in the narrative which becomes more narrative? In this respect, there are two histories of human experience: 1. the stories of the narrative-bound, who perpetrate further narrative, and 2. the record of those who break free from attachment to suffering, either partially or in large measure. One might argue that this latter record is self-dissolving and ultimately invisible. Its practitioners quietly leave the room while the rest of us are struggling, arguing, killing.

Besides, for us as children, and as children of God, this interface is too difficult and complex, and we begin to hope for someone to help us out. The longing for a savior has a superstitious (pigeon) quality—not that a savior wouldn't be nice. In the storm, it is OK to have someone help you from a sinking boat.

In fact, the recognition of an external power within the internal power and enthrallments of personality has some healing potential. Such recognition transcends encapsulation and says, in effect, "As I stand at the door of my house of being, I can look out with hopeful anticipation of recognizing another person, or another portion of self, who is not bad, nor caught in the same way I am, such that he/she is merely mirroring my pattern." For perhaps many, connection with another person at this level is an acknowledged confirmation of direct covenantal connection with God.

At the point or door of our encapsulation, the first person in the world is, like the mother, the savior or messiah. We do not recognize our need for relief from suffering until we sense we are suffering. Because of the difficulty of penetrating the black, we find it almost impossible to acknowledge trauma, and how much our lives are caught and lost in rituals of dissociation. When life comes crashing through these constructs of denial, we are surprised, stunned, and at our worst, establish a commission to look into it. As many have wryly noted, these have come to be known as sins of commission.

Yet as brain discovers its own underlying patternings and begins to find how difficult it is to self-liberate, it appears to develop narrative forms to explain its relationship with the outside world, if it in fact can recognize there is one. In core dissociation, there is no vibrant, relational outside world, nor inner one, for that matter. The ultimate toxicity of traumatic process makes it impossible to garner an adequate and proportioned sense of boundaries, identity, and responsibility. And we look to rules, laws, commandments, guidance, and etiquette, rather than know from within what is appropriate. It is upon this point of recognition that brain says, "Save me."

Salvation

There is no need for saving, for salvation, outside of dissociative process, and yet those who insist no one is exempt from savior mythology are like those therapists who argue for the omnipresence of transference. In most human situations, the phenomena of dissociation appear omni-present and omni-determinate. How foolish of me to say without qualification, in effect, "I am clear of dissociative process," or "I don't need saving." We can well understand the enthusiasm of converts to the faith who try to force people to acknowledge their sinful nature and their need for salvation.

Once dissociation is recognized, the energetic problem is how to reconnect, renegotiate the Covenant, as it were. I think the beginning of the healing process involves brain's recognition of energetic hiatus, held energy, usually occurring in the form of addictive narratives. If we employ narrative, gestalt forms, we turn away from our "self" and look for a savior to clarify how to set the neurochemistry in motion again. The characteristics of our savior will tell us how deeply we understand the mechanism of the traumatic patterning we are in, and to what level or density we are haply, illusorily committed.

If we approach the savior as a politically powerful messiah, one who will lead us out of our oppression, we may get some portion of the patterning out. For example, we shall win the right to vote and to govern ourselves, and perhaps make love with those we love. But if we want full enlightenment, won't we have go deeper than what at least recent politicians have shown us? Our connection must be ultimately with the person standing in front of us, not some generalized, politicized ideal. And in fact, the opportunity to connect, to reestablish the Covenant, is then omnipresent.

Connecting With the Father

Jesus refers to this understanding when he says, in effect, "If you want to connect with the point of origin, the Father, you have to come through me," by which I think he means, "If you don't connect with the incarnate spirit in the form which is in front of you, namely me, or someone else standing before you—the poor, the sinner, whatever—when will you connect? What will it take to reestablish the Covenant? If not now, when?" This strategy-insight often gets instantly transmuted into political rhetoric: "The only way you will get to God is by serving me as your Lord."

If we establish a political relationship of lord and vassal or its equivalent with our dissociative process, what does that say about the healing process? Moreover, how effective a strategy is that for approaching the healing process? Certainly from within traumatic encapsulation, it looks like a savior is the only person or entity who will do the trick.

Savior-seeking can be a position of recognition, a door from the encapsulation of the dissociated process of brain to the outside.

However, in the reworking of held-energy systems, it turns out that something more and less seems required than our dissociative brain estimates. Our brain has more power within than it comprehends and needs to interface more vulnerably with the outside than it has.

For some, invoking the aid of God expresses this understanding, but I favor separating awareness focus away from the risks of savior politics. In the stories of Jesus as healer, he returns the healing power to the individual, in the face of the distraught individual's desire for total, abject rescue. In his company, our healing power is discovered within, the Covenant reestablished again, within.

As with Buddha-consciousness, the way out of suffering may require attentiveness to the self-healing capacity of each individual, not the projection of the miraculous upon an other. Jesus' temptations in the desert as well as his confrontations at the end of his life reflect the danger of assuming such a savior role. If he is a savior, it is a very matter-of-fact, non-exclusive one. It is a role he is prepared share with everyone he meets; and it is no big deal. It is a self-healing energy which he supports in his disciples, and urges them to do likewise: nothing personal.

If we choose a savior as a recognition of our traumatic encapsulation(s), then some healing power appears available Yet how quickly that formulation turns into a service rendered and tempered by ritual and law, not by following the energetic. Our preoccupation becomes with a messiah, not with the power of our own experience.

It has been suggested that over centuries, Jews have hoped for a political solution to this spiritual dilemma, and have sought justice in the world as a way of declaring and serving balance. Yet justice and its implied balance may lapse again into a narrative and retraumatizing formulation, not the essence, and the deepest mystical traditions in Judaism recognize this fact. One hallmark of that lineage has been not naming the Godhead as Source, accurately perceiving its energetic, non-narrative, and invisible nature.

Moses and the Covenant

Because the trauma phenomenon is the central troubling condition of suffering, Jewish lineage gains tremendous focus by the power of the Genesis narrative. It is not hard to imagine how a community which understood the trauma mechanism this well could envision a direct connection to the Godhead in the form of a Covenant. Furthermore, they saw that the Covenant could be socially incarnated.

Most exhaustingly in this regard, the story of Moses contains a vision of the tragic proportions implied in the establishment of the Covenant. Moses sustains witness of the energetic in the bush which burns but is not consumed. More than once, in acts of meditational trust, he goes up upon Mount Sinai to "consult" God, and all sorts of guidance about how to worship, how to construct the temple, what to wear, etc., becomes available to him.

On one occasion of trust on Sinai, the trauma pattern comes up for resolution in the form of the Ten Commandments, which God through Moses has already shared with some of the people Moses has assembled. Moses again needs the Commandments written in stone. While the Ten Commandments help maintain the community and continuity of political religion, their formulation contains an opportunity to abuse the Spirit as well, and we recognize this danger when we caution about something "written in stone."

Jews return to Moses' vision of the burning bush for a description of what the energetic implies, yet Moses encounters the second phase of the trust-trauma sequence and accurately transmits or channels it as commandments set in stone. In the trust of energetic reciprocity, brain offers up for resolution held-energy systems which more than likely have narrative, immobilized form. What may make this sequence so difficult to master is the inner speed of the energetic and its incarnation at the neurochemical level.

Once that level of trust is manifest by Jews as individuals and community, both for Jew and Gentile, the second phase of the mechanism emerges over and over, at both personal and social levels.

Moses breaks the tablets when he sees the people dancing and avoiding the serious, selective spirituality which his Covenant implies. They dig only so far into the problem and, turning their focus away from the spirit, swallow the rest of the banana whole.

A sense of divine "selectivity" is reflected in the idea of being "chosen by God" and, under retraumatization process, appears to become an exclusive and alienating discrimination, from which individuals are excluded. Separation, scapegoating, and mirroring is evoked by those not selected, at all levels, as individuals, and in social, political groups. Most significantly such selectivity may perpetrate division within commonplace, recognizable consciousness, created invisibly by held-energy systems.

Abraham and Isaac

Once the trust phase of the energetic is apprehended as Spirit, it brings forward traumatic patterning in the form of laws and rituals which retraumatize, as well as confuse those particularly dedicated to witnessing and supporting incarnation of the Spirit. The most tragic story of Abraham and Isaac gives shape to the difficulties of generationally transmitting a lineage inspired by insight into the trauma mechanism.

Confusing, and like Merope's, the story of a father about to sacrifice his son reveals how the mechanism shows its radical second-phase, turning within the family, within the self, upon the family and self with awesome subtlety and fearsome speed. And, as Jews point out, in contradistinction to the story of Jesus, which ends in violent death, the story of Abraham and Isaac ends in reconciliation. Yet the narrative of Abraham and Isaac also presents violence, focusing upon the trauma mechanism from an apparently different point of view.

Christians might argue that the death of Jesus also ends in reconciliation with God: a New Covenant announced by Jesus' Resurrection. To enact any full trauma completion, we must go to the site of held-energy, where Jesus is crucified, and the energy appears to be "dead," rather than jumping to the end of the story without describing what the bottoming out, or Crucifixion, looks like. If we ignore the held-energy, we shall merely retraumatize.

All this notwithstanding, both Jews and Christians as groups of people agree on the strategy of what the completing situation must sense like, if not socially, at least, and perhaps most importantly, within personality. Both lineages are concerned with violence and with revising the patterning. In that crucial sense, there is little for Christians and Jews to argue about.

Christians immersed in the ambiance of New Testament revisionism may want to claim that the violence of Jesus' death must be kept in this father-son myth, for the spiritual reconciliation is not yet with us and still needs attending to. Merely not killing the son does not keep the father from perpetrating his patterns. We are still East of Eden.

Jews may invoke the tragic insight that we do not have to see the pattern acted out as Christian tradition has insisted we do. As told, the story of Abraham and Isaac may not get to the point of origin of the perpetrating pattern because its vision of God contains a continual call to obedience, here to the point of a single, strategic sacrifice, rather than to a conclusion of all sacrifice. Christian traditions worry about this in the mythic form of casting the "only begotten son" into an unrescuable immobility, heading directly for the held energy. Both variations are circling the same field, and the disagreements are important and not important.

An ending where there is no sacrifice would take brain out of narrative and out of a hierarchy where one or the other of us, Abraham or Isaac, friend or enemy, Jesus or Pilate, has to channel God's Will. The danger of channelling any Will is wisely noted in both stories. Upon enlightenment, Abraham attends to another of God's angel channels. And Jesus surrenders personal ego-as-channel as he faces death. Jews and Christians both could argue that we have yet to manifest that full energetic, after so short a time: 5,000 or 2,000 years, depending upon where we set down the end of our tape measure.

Jesus and the Trauma Mechanism

The Jewish lineage gains force from the accuracy of its portrait in Genesis of infantile development as well as from its intuitive command of the issues surrounding the trauma mechanism. At its worst, like every lineage, the revelation of the patterns and the energy released within them leads to perpetrations, against themselves collectively as well as directing the abuse outward in the form of rigid and restrictive boundarying.

Not being chosen is nothing new, nor exclusive to Jews. What might be particularly painful for Jews collectively may be the confounding thwarting of eros which as a group they confront in the world. Though their mythic fingers have been on the pulse of suffering's source, often they have been powerless to reduce it.

With the emergence of the figure of Jesus or the lineage of community, probably Essene, which he has come to characterize, a regaining of connection to the energetic appears manifest at the periphery of a retraumatizing phase of Jewish lineage, even to the point of the so-called miraculous. Over centuries, the crisis of authority which Jews have generated with their understanding of the trauma mechanism, and its resultant hope for Covenental relationship with God, is in Jesus again addressed with his focusing upon the same mechanism.

Christian lineage challenges the retraumatizations by the Old Testament social structures which were designed to preserve focus on the identical territory which, if it were known, is the precious focus of both political religions. These lineages, Jews and Gentiles, become increasingly self-characterizing as different, to the point of long-term illusory disputation and not illusory persecution.

Over centuries, the focus upon the trauma mechanism breeds not only a sense of balance, often promulgating conversion, liberation, and enlightenment. It evokes within and without the communities of the New Testament traumatic patternings and attempts to master these patterns through retraumatizing activities.

Classical social order seems transformed only to be confronted immediately with the second stage of the trauma mechanism, namely the next held-energy system coming up for resolution. Because this shows up usually in its most difficult, "impossible" form, offered by the brain suddenly, without preamble, it often has been impossible to see the victim hiding within the perpetrator, or vice versa.

Christians and Jews

As a community and as a group, Jews come to experience how Christian insight and so-called transformation rarely leads to a situation of trust so much as it does to perpetration of the Christian lineage of traumatic abuse, usually predicated within the Christian hope of healing.   If Christians have hoped for conversion for everyone, haven't Jews watched for the second shoe?

As victims caught in a victim/perpetrator vortex, Jews have learned the complexity of this trauma mechanism, though they seemed powerless to rework it in a favor which could be called theirs, or bring it to successful completion. As a result, and predicted in the outlines of Genesis, the Jewish, and neo-Jewish, *i.e.*, Christian, lineage of sacred eros is truncated in a confounding and ethnically perpetuated series of activities which often appear to take the believer further away from Covenant with the Godhead, not closer, as s/he fervently desires.

The Christian reidentifying of the trauma mechanism promises to restore a vision of the energetic which is sacred, personal, erotic, sensately relational, and compassionate, a vision which at crucial points in our experience the traumatized so-called Christian mindbody cannot find nor sustain.   Nor can the desired realization be superimposed or feigned, as many of us attempt to do, through etiquette, morality, law, and ethical behavior.   In order to be sustainable and significant, discovery of the light appears to have to come as of something out of nothing, facing as it were, the blackest place, in the energetic company of another being, "where two or three are gathered."

We do need a savior, if by saying that, we are recognizing the need for the experience of a reciprocally oscillating human energetic field, within and without personality patterning. Then the held-energy systems can be reworked, and are, with relative ease, given the magnitude of the problem as the brain initially perceives it, and as brain holds on to it, often for decades and often to the death. But again, how instantaneously that messiah can become politicized and sadistically elaborated, as in the configuration of the Crucifixion.

Jesus, Buddha, the oriental masters, and other avatars reiterate that the savior comes in any form, in any guise, that the hunt for a rescuing messiah, while understandable, is beside the point. Our salvation from the wages of held-energy systems can mean allowing brain to rework the information at a subtle energy level at least, invisible to the machinations of ordinary consciousness.

Where we address the mystery through the energetic, we can get a feel for our powers to heal ourselves. That we may need the palpable presence of another person to achieve this knowledge at the deepest levels seems a kind of graceful, connecting, cozy fact of life. That this condition has been so often obscured may have to do with political as well as personal and energetic reasons.

The Need for a Messiah

A main difficulty for Jews as a collective with political Christianity seems to be the idolatry which surrounds Jesus. The commonplace attitude appears as, "I don't think Jesus is the Messiah." But when have you heard in theological debate between Christians and Jews, who surely have reason for concern, a discussion about why is there a need for a messiah, or what are the dangers implicit in guru worship?

Why does it appear that historically Jews have focused upon saying Jesus is not the Messiah, representing themselves as disregarding the wisdom of what Jesus said about the Spirit, much of which has been presaged in the Jewish prophetic lineage? Why is the fight about messiah-ship, rather than about the pitfalls which arise from *any* political resolution to spiritual clarification?   The "arguments" on both sides often appear to me to reveal a shallowness of spiritual understanding perpetrated within both lineages.

Jews can object to the hypocrisy that political Christianity engenders, with its surprising and unsurprising abusive patterns against the Jews, as well as fellow Christians, which puts the lie to the embodiment of espoused Christian faith. Yet in their own certainty, Jews and Christians, speaking collectively, might miss the point of the message of one from within Jewish lineage, namely that just around the corner, a new Covenant with God, the Kingdom of God, awaits everyone, within each one of us. By politicizing religion, by imposing dogmatics and dogmatic personality style upon the Spirit, what is valuable in the Jewish tradition becomes a rigidity which invites overthrow, by Jews and Christians alike.

Christians, inspired by the vision of freedom implied in Jesus' revision of Torah authoritarianism, can feel threatened by that rigidity in Jewish lineage, and invite them by conversion, as it were, out of the cold into the hot tub of affiliation and forgiveness. Yet for the most part, when encountering the objections of Jews to Christ Jesus worship, Christians become defensive, "unChristian," unresponsive, dissociative, and abusive, proving again that their initial reaching out to Jews is false, or problematically framed. If Jesus is the Messiah, He has not prevented abuses among his believers. The real Messiah is yet to come.

While the simple message about any messiah strategy implies a place of vulnerability, wherein we need to be saved, or, originally, ruled by an anointed one, our focus on the nature of the messiah again determines what we are being saved from, or about.   Or more remarkably, what we *think* we are being saved from or about. And even more ironically, whether we can choose who that messiah will be, or which one we shall give our allegiance to, as if, from an absurdist perspective, that might make an ultimate difference. Of course, our choice, if it could be called that, of messiah profile will tell us a lot about where in relation to traumatic process we are positioned.

The simple Christian insight and one that many Jewish thinkers have registered, but more popularly since Freud, is that the healing capacity is within everyone, and can be manifest from even the most abject of places in our personality. In fact those appear to be the starting places of discovery offered by brain for its own pattern unravelling.

Yet even when he speaks of coming to the Father through him, I think Jesus has to be read carefully. It is easy to drive beyond the exit of what he is saying. What appears most matter-of-fact is that if you are going to break the pattern, and achieve enlightenment, it will take place within the context of an ordinary man who, for lack of a better term, hovers with what we have called clear life energy, not any king or political religionist, or religious politico. To achieve that, we must pay attention to our own experience of held-energy systems, not to someone else's.

Jesus Dies For Our Sins

To say that the Messiah has come and has done what is necessary for a messiah to do can mean that someone has acknowledged the Godhead within him/herself, and that that particular destiny does not have to be destructively enacted or reenacted. We do not have to repeat our infantile, traumatically skewed grandiosity. It can be dropped. We thus place ourselves in a radical new historical neurochemistry, one closer, hopefully, to the center of our trauma, wherein there was no savior nor messiah besides the trauma mechanism itself.

As part of traumatic patterning, the experience stated in the Crucifixion has been accomplished already within us, and it can best be approached as in fact it has been laid in, as something which is historically in the past, and in a sense, beyond time. Developmentally, we are traumatized already, and the Crucifixion states its nature as being within held energy.

In the distortions and grandiosity of scale engendered by trauma (*cf.* the only "Only Begotten Son"), to experience Crucifixion again merely would be retraumatization. This is one way to approach the chemistry expressed by "Jesus died for our sins." The story of Jesus' death describes our traumata and their held-energy systems, including its necessity for self-completion from the most difficult place of immobility, here (on) the Cross. Within a similar perspective about retraumatization, the Second Coming may describe our entry into the held-energy system for final resolution of the traumatic pattern, from and at T-*zero* [T_0].

CHAPTER EIGHT: CHRISTIANS AND JEWS

Chosen

Another meaning behind messianic concerns is that the Christ energy can be manifest at every point. In fact that may be the only way for us to keep clear. Obviously, anybody can manifest Christ energy particularly, including Jews. Jesus himself incarnates the Christ energy, or its vibration level. It could be argued that as a Jew he also channels it, even though the presence of that energy invites the emergence of held-energy systems within his proximity.

This high vibration, non-denominational energy evokes the split, the dissociation, perhaps accounting for the dividuation between Christians and Jews, Jews and Jews, Christians and Christians, and everyone else in the world, particularly those who determine their identity through ethnic and religious affiliations. As individuals outside these religious groupings, we may be abandoned to conduct our own spiritual journey, isolated, invisible, and unrecognized.

Jews as a group with a collective identity and experience know of the Christ energy when they embody their special Covenant with God, reflected in the emotional narrative that they can feel chosen. In a private, unsticky formulation, feeling chosen can mean balanced, integrated, connected living.

However, the focus upon feeling chosen may include traps of consolidation around a fate which fosters abandonment, envy, and persecution, and their compensations. These are "temptations" which Jesus experiences. And for the individual who pursues that fate, whether card-carrying Christian or Jew, the abusive pattern continues, generated by invisible held-energy systems, with nothing learned.

Sustaining the neurochemistry of the Christ energy implied in the Covenant is apparently not fully, socially understood within the Jewish lineage until the centuries immediately preceding Jesus, because the energetic is not embodied yet in a comprehensive mimetic gestalt. Jesus, particularly for Christians, appears to be such a gestalt of Old Testament heroic, tragic conundra, rendered into the narrative of a single personality.

In their political religiosity, Christians, again considered as a collective identity, have the support as do Jews of ethical systems supposedly in place to protect them from making errors. But those systems generally do not keep them from making errors. Thus, we ask, is some deeper pattern at work and not within social control?

These violations, or mistakes, are encapsulations of energy which can reflect misunderstandings of reality as it could be if we live at the highest vibrational levels. When embodied, Christ energy liberates not as a result of mere revisions to the Ten Commandments but because of a process neurochemical and prior to addictive behavior, traumatically determined. Like its early form, the burning bush, it moves through and within forms which threaten to betray its essence, beyond political religion and ethnic identity.

Who is Christian?

Who then is Christian? Is that different from being Jewish? Are there significant differences in actual life experience between ordinary Christians and Jews? There may be two kinds of experience to focus upon: the true Christ energy, and the identity of the political Christian, who does not or only partially manifests Christ energy. Both modes include registered Jews and Christians alike and, I think, cannot be distinguished except by careful intuition, not just by our outside behavior nor, for that matter, when viewed from within.

It seems our soul observes itself in its hapless imprisonment of the body and culture into which it may choose to be born. Does this imprisonment determine the states of realization of its true nature? In this, spiritual Christian experience may mirror Buddha consciousness, perhaps with similar vibrational levels, with similar tasks to reduce the dualism inherent in our traumatic process.

Traditionally, the same problem is addressed from similar phases. The Buddhist seeks enlightenment and the end of suffering. The Christian seeks salvation, the restoration of Covenental relationship with God and the conclusion of suffering, while the Jew seeks restoration of the Covenant and wholeness through just relationship with God and fellow man—concluding our suffering.

It may be important to reiterate that I refer to those aspects of individuals who choose identifications based upon religious and ethnic belief systems and associations. Exceptions aside, most of us reside at these levels, or revert to them when we are anxious. I think private spirituality—direct knowledge of the Spirit—remains more private and not easily available to public examination or to even private self-examination, because of dissociation.

Energy and Former Lives

The influence of ideas and doctrine on our perception of the energetic can be profound. What is the nature of a disturbing idea? Is it disturbing because it brings challenges the brain cannot absorb? Or make sense of? Or because such ideas remind us that we don't understand this universe?

Why, for example, is reincarnation declared heretical to the canon of classical Catholic Christianity? Its elimination appears to remove a complex sense of placement in time which has the potential for encouraging psychodynamic fuzziness. In our current fashionable immersion in reincarnation strategies, we know now again how the assimilation of an idea idiosyncratically percolates.

Coming from a position of the aftershocks of pagan and Judeo-classical excesses, to be told you are living in a present where so-called Jesus is resurrected and is here and now, or coming again soon, brings an immediacy to the idea of the Holy Spirit, the energy, which is hopeful and transforming. The disturbing idea of resurrection takes us up close to reincarnation, and, I think, to the structure and fate of held-energy systems.

To have to wait lifetimes, or to defer the confrontation with the Ultimate until an other life after this one seems cruel and abusive, and to support prolonged denial, which is not what Jesus, for one, appeared to be about. Under reincarnation rubrics, the social order can go to hell in a basket before streets are tidied up and starving children fed, same as here.

Perhaps the chronic misuse of the reincarnation strategy proves offensive, or its champions become politically inconvenient to some bishop or interest group at the Second Council of Constantinople in 553 A.D. when reincarnation is declared heretical. Yet it could be argued that reincarnation and associated karmic strategies, ancient and profound, have been preserved by the Roman Catholic Church in concealed forms. The doctrines of the Resurrection of the Body, Life after Death, the Second Coming, and the concept of Original Sin, among others, appear as gerrymandered, journeyman renderings, with little of the lightness, humor, and deftness which the most skillful use of these more ancient strategies invites and requires.

We have only to enter one of our current healing networks in America to see how idea-insight systems like reincarnation must have floated throughout what is now the Middle East. We can see in our fads and new therapies how Eastern ideas could get absorbed into the Christian dogma.

But with reincarnation, in the sixth century, some line appears drawn and not crossed, except daily in these above-mentioned doctrines, altered forms wherein the implications cannot be evaluated, because the healing context of the ideas has been removed or muted. Only now it seems possible in the West to use the strategy to return literally not to what is imaginatively known about, say, previous lives, but to see it as a graceful road to mystery, enlightenment—beyond former lives and into the energetic.

Over centuries, the treatment of the mentally ill has rarely succeeded. These days, the hope for medication to transform personality is possible to maintain, yet for ill and well alike, our ultimate patterning experience can be that of pattern removal, not merely pattern clarification, adjustment, suppression, and accommodation. What medication takes us to is considering ourselves neurochemically, and beyond that, energetically.

In the Eastern strategies surrounding incarnation and karma, we also witness centuries-old patterns coming into mindbodies in order to be resolved. In a held-energy sense, karma equals trauma, the opportunity to experience and watch the pattern dissolve. With Buddhism, we are offered a vision of Nirvana wherein ego, based upon held-energy systems, does not exist, and where what is, is seen as OK. From this position, violence is not tolerated nor sought.

I find it interesting that, whereas Buddhist lineages suggest with enlightenment an end of suffering, the (Judeo-)Christian lineage offers salvation through a specific image which depicts the cruciform suffering incarnation of held energy. Both are attending to the perpetrating instrumentation of the held-energy systematics from various points in the trauma sequence, the Christian modality tracing down the impact of trauma as we embody it.

In the Buddhist tradition, if there is a final, heavenly resort, it involves the clearing out of ego. In the Christian and Jewish lineages at their most subtle, there is no ego. Short of that, there is political religion, forced and forcing people into compliance with political and social orders, many of which seem absolutely necessary to public order and decency.

But most lineages do not take us actively past their doctrines, their rigidities, to the place beyond doctrine. And they argue that we cannot go there because to do that would be to remove all meaning and structure, to invite chaos. Yet that is precisely the point. To *not* perpetrate the patterns—the lineages of abuse—is, I think, as difficult and worthwhile a beachhead to land on and stake a flag, as did any colonizing child of the Renaissance placing a cross in the sand of the

New World. And in addition to a Christian vision of freedom, we
know what other patterns these European children rendered.

More on Christians and Jews

Christians, grounded in the myth of Genesis, somehow
experience the centrality of the Christ energy. Yet by characterizing
it with exclusivity in the figure of Jesus, they may reflect dissociate
process, as do Jews who read "chosen" as "the only ones who are
chosen." Yet the chemistry of held-energy systems can be entered,
perhaps only, from that chosen, only begotten position.

In the dissociative spiritual practice of the traumatized
(Christian) brain, once sensing the energetic trust, Christians
historically have offered up their traumata, for healing, only not really.
Their offering looks more like the religious wars following the
Reformation. This partial resolution gives their faith the lie.

Jews and Protestants may have glanced at each other to see
how to coexist here in the "Catholic" West in spite of both groups
standing outside the self-proclaiming, established center of
Catholicism. As self-establishing center, might Catholicism itself be
seen as a revolt against the stone-like anti-spiritualism of Jews,
Gentiles, and others—those a revolt against the randomness of desert
cults and faiths?

Each political Christian can be seen as a partial Christian,
because his/her identity depends upon a social and political alignment
with perpetrative communal forms. Most Christians admit this partial
mastery, but few will give up Jesus, or the idea of this Christ, Jesus,
as just one more attachment to another Jew, or hero, or guru. But at
the center of our experience, I sense trauma determines most of our
activity and thinking, and at the center of trauma is held, Christ,
energy, not its "perfect" incarnation.

Jews as group and individuals have come to be rightly wary,
skeptical, even paranoid of self-stylized Christians who have had
access to this transforming of consciousness, of time and personality.

Like Jews themselves, these Christians may not acknowledge the second phase of a lineage of generations of political, social, personal and intrapsychic abuse, except in the name of Christianity to act it out, in discrimination, pogroms, and holocausts, as perpetrator and/or victim.

If individual Jews ask themselves why, as souls, they have incarnated as Jews in this lifetime, have taken on such a burden, the answer, I think, must be what has always been the task for people as Jews, to see if they can let the patterns dissolve, to reestablish the energetic Covenant from that position of exile. In this objective, they are, of course, like us all, hidden saints, taking up an ethnic burden which has itself taken up the burden of humanity, to solve the problem contained in the trauma mechanism, first explicated, and rightly placed first, in the Garden of Eden. How close to "solving" the conundrum of trauma are we? Can we witness it at its energetic levels?

Jews and Protestants

The Protestant is a small movement, perhaps a fraction of the total humanoid configuration of energy and trauma, but, I think, not one to be dismissed. Protestants and Jews share more than they think. They share a dislike of what is rigid and authoritarian, yet in their polymorphism, their diversity, they may reflect certain pivotal rigidities which are retraumatizing. Many Jews say they honor freedom, yet at racial, ethnic levels, with humor, they can express feeling stuck at "being" Jews.

By disavowing an energetic lineage, where major figures such as Moses and the prophets perceived the truth as individuals, they may perpetrate a social order like any other, which haplessly can draw them away from Covenant, as individuals as well as an ethnic community. Their collective desires for security through power seem as fragile and hapless as the Christians', or anyone else's.

As a lineage, Protestants appear stuck standing against authority, a defense that hopes to generate movement within held-energy systems in the authority by retraumatizing, by reenacting the trauma. The view of history from this perspective is rarefied. In each configuration of sectional belief, Jew, Protestant, and Catholic, the held-energy systems appear to be in competition for resolution, like rivalrous siblings demanding undivided attention from a harried mother.

The Protestant Movement

With the Renaissance and the Protestant Reformation, the focus on the trauma mechanism called Christianity might fall roughly into three "post-Jewish" modalities, the Catholic, the Protestant, and the humanistic-scientific. In each mode, the nature of authority is challenged because of retraumatizing perpetrations by the very institutions and individuals declared to defend the Faith. The faith includes a vision of held-energy systems, as well as a recognition that we cannot alleviate our suffering by direct, simple, willful intention ("Just make it better.").

Furthermore, these modes prepare for the emergence of further levels of traumatic experience generated by the trust these forms have achieved. In the all-too-predictable representative case of the protestant Luther, he eventually becomes the punitive, perpetrative authority he once challenged.

The Protestant heritage has yet to be fully acknowledged, particularly by current Protestants themselves. Historically, the Protestant movement breaks the gridlock of Catholic, patristic authoritarianism, so-called, and separates out into a series of fractionating communities clustering around belief systems, some mirroring, some refracting, some individuating from external, and gradually from internal, psychological authoritarianism. Each progression of Protestantism yields a more visible picture of the nature of the held-energy beast, actually a process, and of how to resolve its toxic effects within society and within the soul of man.

A basic question all three political religious modes ask is "From where within the psyche does authority gain its allegiance?" I suggest that the authority each attempts to redefine rests within the invisibility of the experience of traumatic process, both its negative and positive aspects. In Protestantism we may see a reworking of the territory first identified and described by Jews in Genesis and later encompassed within original sin strategies, and reflects a partial understanding of held-energy systems, which carry an ultimate authority in our neurochemistry.

For Original Sinners, authority is declared and confronted in the episode of eating of the apple, perhaps imitating a birth process, wherein the traumatic past is stored and memorized. We are separated into fractional consciousness, not by opposition to God, or by disobedience, which I take to be elaborations by the mindbody upon its confounding inability to penetrate the neurochemical gates of held energy. Rather, we are separated by the process in primitive brain which is designed to protect us in times of crisis. As healers in the Jewish and Christian traditions suggest, evil is nothing more than held energy, incompletely understood by its "containers."

While the axis of trust and trauma is for the most part accurately described in Genesis, it is important to note that the story is told to and from the traumatized portions or levels of brain, not to the fully liberated, de- or untraumatized ones. When Luther claims his own right and necessity to interpret the Bible, he protests against the sacerdotal immobility of the Catholic Church and toward a reconnection with the energetic. He is like the child no longer needing its mother's sacerdotal function as interpreter of reality: "That's all right, we can get another ice cream cone to replace the one you have dropped and are incorrectly mourning as if this were the end of the world."

Yet Luther's stand is taken within retraumatizing institutions of language and emerging national identity. He does not challenge the Bible, but rather the Pope's right to exclusively interpret it. The sequencing of trust and trauma suggests that the original Eden as a place of trust is bound to provoke the appearance of any residual trauma latent in the psyche. After Wittenburg it does, with lots of lengthy killing and traumatizing violence. Over centuries, the trauma patterning in Europe is only slowly approached both for individuals and for social groups, reemerging periodically for final solutions.

As a political collective, Catholics may be of small help to the Jews, even though they themselves are in revolt against held-energy systems, as well as the social, personal, and political traumata these systems contain. They personally and collectively may abandon the Jew who may perpetrate a lineage of abuse, as perpetrator and/or victim, just as Catholics are also abandoned by the establishment and maintenance of a Church hierarchy which denies, distrusts, subverts, and intrudes upon the sacred eros of its members. The lineage of abuse continues through the hapless flounderings of perpetrator and victim, all victims alike.

At the heart of Protestantism, and its handmaiden, democracy, is the realization that any authority is challengeable. Authoritarianism, wherein authority demands allegiance merely because it is authority, is recognized as abusive. Various sects develop which replace the old tyrannies with new ones. Yet, as a function of the trust-trauma axis, few in each sect appear able to evoke a vision of trauma-free energy during which the trauma phase of the trust-trauma sequence is not fervently offered up, for healing, of course, though it looks like perpetration. I think it is the difficulty of holding on to this sustained vision which leads to Adventist, Second Coming, and end-of-the-world elaborations. These belief systems promise a new, non-traumatizing reckoning.

The *protestant* movement is not over. Its implications are still playing themselves out in dramatic and compelling forms. Most significantly, I think, is the deepening challenge to the sacerdotal function of authority. If authority stands between us and our sensate experience as individuals, we are vulnerable to splitting, domination, and loss of integrity. There is a valuable reinforcement for Jews from the protestant experience, and I think it has to do with issues raised by the figure of Moses.

As a leader who stands against the authority of Pharaoh, Moses acts sacerdotally, interpreting and connecting for his people, but we do not see how he approaches the energetic. We merely see the results, in the form of social limit-setting and perhaps obsessional elaborations. He does not invite us to see the bush with him. Like an imperceptive analyst, doesn't he present the results, in the form of fiat interpretations, rather than letting us see the bush for ourselves?

A central potency of the Protestant Reformation is the call again to experience direct Covenant with God, within existing social orders and without. This focus meets Jews as a mythic identity where they have been stuck, which may in part account for distrust between Jews and Protestants. This is a ram's horn call which has alerted Jews through the centuries, the call to worship, but not to experience the very same patterning which Jews resist in the deadened faith of so many contemporary Protestants. The radical experience of taking a risk at this personal level is something which has been recorded in Holocaust literature, where individual stories of courage and enlightenment have been lived and experienced under a black held-energy system whose anti-vibrational after-shocks are still paradoxically reverberating.

For Jews and Christians, Protestant and Catholic, the demanding and ambivalating tyranny of held-energy systems is, I suspect, the authority which we all are protesting against and within, not so-called political and religious tyrannies which imitate their serious, even deadly (in)action. That the trauma mechanism has been energetically concealed, but the effects of its perpetrative manifestation disastrously have not been, is a human sadness and waste hard to encompass.

The Tyranny of Traumatic Patterning

Why does it take us so long to remove traumatic patterning? These patterns are held at an invisible, black, level, which is neuro-chemically fended from brain's ordinary capacity to solve the chemical hiatus. Black nexuses of energy evolve throughout the personality, often spindling on a primal trauma, either directly transmitted by violence, or indirectly transmitted by personality osmosis, mirroring, or "education." Things go fine until pockets of suffering suddenly emerge, or we find ourselves conspiring with someone else to declare each other enemies.

I intuit that these systems of held energy then provide pivots for behavior and so-called personality, that the axis of what we recognize about personality reveals not an open set of choices, but reflects what our brain has done with held energy. Various spatiousnesses are tracked in, but as with the creation of arable land by building the dikes of Holland, always there is the threat that the basic alignment of these held-energy systems may be shifted or taken away.

That these held-energy systems in themselves are based on illusion, the illusion that we are still in trauma-inducing situations when we are not, is of course confounding. Brain appears to appropriate the information contained in the held-energy system instantly, usually without time to process it in tranquil recollection. It takes on messages which are important, but they are not placed historically in their proper, for lack of a better term, historical perspective.

We then must identify where they are located and under what conditions they are laid in, not quite the same as recreating the narrative. Eleanor is gasping for breath, reporting, "I cannot breathe," yet, in a wobbly fashion, she is breathing. She has to wait at the neurochemical interface between traumatic past and current present until brain resolves the crisis.

At the core of the held-energy system is a pattern which can self-dissolve, restoring mobility and flexibility which we can experience as clear. Ethnicities, personality fragments, and organizations appear to fall short of clear, so-called choice.

The sad but necessary sequence seems to be that once we achieve some higher vibrational state, other fragments in the self begin to appear to seek completion. Or from the outside, people volunteer and perpetrate their trauma upon our momentarily clearer and not necessarily fully sustained vibrational condition. I think this is what may have happened in the complex case of Jesus' death: *nothing personal.*

CHAPTER NINE: CHRIST-ENERGY AND AUTHORITY

The Life Energy

Why is any of this religious lineage important? First of all, the specific forms which I am considering here are mythic variations of ethnic and religious patterning, and themselves represent universal themes. Furthermore, I am considering group identities which are variable and for which personal exceptions always may be a rule. We cannot speak of all Jews or all Catholics or all Protestants and expect the discussion to move very realistically. It would be most accurate perhaps to say none of the generalizations stated herein really apply to you, reader.

But patterning at this group level does exist, and people are responsive to those formulations and social pressures for identity, recognizability, and communication. At some level, however, these generalizations can reveal the essential problem of how narrative patterns are passed on in lineages of instruction. So identifying the interface of these cultural bumper cars may be fruitful for seeing how the patterning can be changed by locating where it begins. We may know that Monet creates or causes the painting, but when we are viewing it, we need to know that our witnessing of it begins where it is hung in Gallery A.

Religious lineages can reveal spiritual vectors and their distortions, which, I propose, can help us to see these beginnings. To find the origin of movement, can we discover the origin of traumata and recognize when people as individuals or as parts of groups are in various stages of toxicity from their effects? My clients and I have sensed that no movement, psychic or otherwise, is considered real or non-compensatory by brain unless the underlying traumatic patterning has been dissolved.

Over time in the West, examinations of life energy, the energetic, have been dominated by the life and experience of Jesus: Christ. While some might characterize our understanding of the life energy essentially as Christ energy, I see problems that overlap with its mythic embodiment in the life of Jesus, which I shall try to enumerate. Furthermore, I think the Christ energy is not merely a (the) manifestation of clear life energy, but, as elaborated in the West, it includes its held-energy form as well.

Both the Reformation and scientific revolution rework the sacerdotal question, namely, can we communicate with God directly, or do we need mediation? Against our experience of religious fanaticism in ourselves and others, which has perpetrated social and personal catastrophe, collective wisdom suggests mediational intervention, agreement, and dialogue. Against our experience of the violations of mediational trust, the turning of that trust into pernicious and lethal monkey business suggests the risks of giving over our responsibility to someone else.

Both tails of this sacerdotal question wag from the dog of dissociation, again reflecting the power of our held-energy systems to distort and confound. Historically, since the Reformation we have established new strategies for approaching all levels of experience, including authority and the energetic. Increasingly the traditional Gospels are challenged about their inconsistencies, their irrealism, as well as the essential truth which they convey. The mythic truths and values are separated from the individual who inspires the movement called Christianity, and after centuries, it becomes permissible to ask who the real man, Jesus, was, or is.

In its current form, the search for the historical Jesus, the man in and beyond the myth, goes back at least 150 years, though we might claim it has always been present, since the time he lived. Within this scholarly attempt to identify who Jesus really was and what he actually said and did, is, I think, an attempt to see the Godhead directly. This is preferable to viewing Gospel encrustations of superstitious response to the impenetrability of (some, important) black.

The identification of the historical Jesus is a contemporary reworking of the earlier preoccupations, among others, with the covering of Jesus' genitalia in Renaissance paintings, where the Holy Spirit was witnessed as directly incarnate, unavoidably human, and lineage-based (cf. Steinberg). Yet to claim Jesus as the exclusive clear transmitter of this so-called life energy may be a misapplication, counter-productive, limiting, and, in its current formulations associated with the life of Jesus as presented in the Gospels, I believe, it has proven dangerous. Clerics who wrestle with interpretation of text every week in their homilies fight this fight.

One reason why the focus has been on Jesus, rather than each one of us, has been to keep the laity safe by projecting our understanding and capacities onto a suitable representation, a *mimēsis*, of our essential selves. The best reason for not witnessing the clear energetic in each individual is to protect us from a totality of sensate experience which is not supported in our community. Even more, it is actively crushed as the trauma mechanism in our surround is evoked by the vibrational trust the clear energy conveys; *nothing personal*. As with David Karesh, uncovering it in the lay person may lead to expression not only of the energetic but of its held, demonic, even abusive forms, both in the individual and in the accommodation of the mirroring, completing social environment.

Who is the Christ?

As we uncover the historical man Jesus, we also discover the "historical" Christ, an important mythic proposition about self which dovetails and interweaves with the probable life of a Jew, an Essene?, 2,000 years ago. Who or what is the Christ and what does he/she/it look like and feel?

While Christology as a term appears to occur first in English in the mid-seventeenth century, the study of the nature of the Christ predates Jesus and finds resonances even today in our continuing search for individuals who manifest wholeness, the balanced, integrated, self-realized, fully-developed presence of the essential Godhead, the person who sustains clear Covenant with ultimate reality. I think this being is not the same as the becoming of a messiah, though it can be a commentary upon messianism.

Pre-Christian Hellenic traditions steeped in tragedy and tragic theory encompassed approaches to scapegoating from projective patterns involving our understanding of ourselves as hero. Our insights about what the Christ is seem to have to do with finding a human, gestalt imitation or representation of the energetics of trauma embedded in the heroic. This mimetic encompasses a portrait of the savior hero-god who will die and resurrect, itself a narrative *mimēsis* of what happens energetically when brain moves neurochemically from held and formal narrative immobility to energetic, invisible mobility.

In dissociation, the relationships between inside and outside, private and public, individual and politically social are often distorted. They await recalibration. That the Christ energy ultimately resides not at the social, but at the individual level appears strategic to heroic positioning. The heroic mode simultaneously also expresses the hyperbolic compression of life energy in held-energy systems, as each of us carries them.

Thus ideas about crucifixion, death, and resurrection are not necessarily fanciful denials of people who cannot rationally face death. They can communicate the nature of the direct, inner experience of trauma resolution. This is important, Good News.

Historically, this understanding of trauma resolution appears superimposed by his followers upon the stories and sayings of Jesus, who as a person apparently presented as remarkably *clear*. Many people now suggest not only was he clear as a child but also was enhanced in this clarity as a young adult studying and practicing yogic, meditational healing traditions in India and the Far East.

In the mix of subsequent religious and social upheavals, his strategies and commentaries for life are developed as followers try to find the cause, then the initiating point of suffering evoked, perhaps exemplified by his clarity. What we can discover in the *muthos* of Jesus' life is that the presenting, evoking cause of suffering is not the initiating point (T_0) of the pattern of suffering, and he is in fact fully "innocent." *Nothing personal.*

The formulations about the Christ ultimately reside within the energetic, often so-called mystical, realms, and certainly are invisible to ordinary— *i.e.*, dissociative— consciousness. Our concerns about the nature of the Christ focus upon how the subtle energetic is understood and brought into ordinary life—in short, incarnated. If we need a savior, a messiah, then he/she/it must be something like a Christ. Nothing less will do, because we intuit that the Christ function entails the held-energy system, black child of trauma, as well as the memory of experience before its installation, and our anticipation of its resolution.

Jesus on the Cross

As the Christ lineage has been exclusively appropriated by some followers of Jesus, as contrasted, say, with the followers of some Dionysian cult with similar resurrection formulations, one of our main images of the incarnated Christ energy is that of Jesus dying on the Cross. In art, literature, music, drama, and theology, this is the end point of reference for all depictions of Jesus' earlier life, from the Annunciation on. As Reich has also seen, this image provides an entry into unravelling not only what dissociative process looks like, but what Christ energy, if you will, involves. For it contains the familiar, characteristic two-phase, perhaps contradictory, certainly alternating sequencing of the trauma mechanism.

Traumatic in nature, the crucifixion image can be seen as a description of brain's early approach into the black of held-energy, and brain's strategy for appropriating the information within these systems being delivered to it. Even more specifically, trauma thus depicted resides in the verticality and horizontality of the spinal "aura" or energetic. Furthermore, if I were asked what does the approach to held energy look like within the neurochemistry, to the neurochemistry of trauma, the Cross would be a crucial example.

In the rigid, wooden Cross, there is no energetic movement, and the mindbody suffers its narrative position, held and unapproachable, a paradigm of dissociation, whose point of origin cannot be seen. The subsequent, critical experience of watching the held energy transform into movement, even ultimately into play—Glory—is only later demonstrated theologically in Jesus' story by his Ascension. My friend Timothy Sens considers the Crucifixion a distraction from this more central action, and I understand his point.

By keeping the clearest vibrational levels away from common access, or by setting it exclusively as a Christ against a Cross of unnecessary and brutal victimization performed 2,000 years ago, do we not focus on and perpetuate a solution of political density? This configuration, with its concomitant and associated dangers of violence and sentimentality, holds only a hint of resolution of the pattern, and an incomplete *mimēsis* of the way through.

The form of a cross, with its juxtaposed right angle vectors, is often at the center of trauma energetics and their resolution As with vampire "tamers," the cross might be "held up" in the face of demonic elaboration to still that process, because these juxtaposing vectors are what seems to trouble brain. Or they "hold" our pre-windshield chaos in a dominant, but ultimately false stability.

The cross is a potent symbol of the energetic crux which must self-dissolve. We would never want it out of our energetic toolbox (do we have a choice?), and in many cases, it is a primary form in which patterns ultimately show up for completion. Yet while it may describe a phase of most trauma resolution, it is not the only form amid which suffering is experienced or relieved.

Two Phases to the Christ Energy

The figure of Jesus on the Cross can be seen to have two main contradictory yet crucially related phases, vis-à-vis traumatic patterning. The first is of energetic immobility, a representation of life energy held in, nailed to, traumatic patterning. This is the energy which carries with it the heroic, grandiose elaboration of the Savior, the Messiah, who takes away the sins of the world. It mimics the hyperbole of dissociated neurochemistry, as well as a factual characteristic of clear life energy. This is part of what people think of when they define the Christ as Jesus on the Cross. It is This One who will save them.

The second phase is the transition out of trauma, including the implied Resurrection, and Ascension, which portrays a dropping off of virtually all patterning, consistent with Buddhist detachment. That crucifixion imagery only suggests a restoration of a fluid, non-Messianic, post-Christ integrity may be because our immersion into the energetic means a giving up of all forms, which in language and art may be very hard to convey.

For our so-called personalities, we are not unlike pinballs bumping against the numbered posts of held-energy systems within our neurochemistries. Because we cannot enter them, and they seem solid, we bounce against them in the mistaken awareness that as immobilities, they are what is solid within us. At their core, these "bumpers" are clear, energetic, and dissoluable. Paradoxically, when these posts of held energy are removed, we may experience a deeper, truer freedom than we have thought we wanted or can easily tolerate.

Though pervasive, and an initial step toward acknowledging suffering, the desire for a messiah may be thus beside the point, not because there have not been successful implementations of this strategy in exceptional miraculous healing—all healing is miraculous—nor because they have seemed so rare. And some might argue that they are not rare but are omnipresent. To seek lifting off the patterning by someone outside ourselves in the form of a splinter-removing Savior, while OK, may distract us from finding the healing power of our brain's own energetic.

Perhaps this strategy was never really offered in the way I am suggesting. How do we envision spirit within personality? One common approach sets God the Spirit politically above ordinary human concerns, connected with some sinful state or predicament which then is incarnated and transformed.

Can we move between the two phases of life energy, the traumatically impacted and the integrated, to perceive our preoccupation with the so-called Christ and the form we have chosen, accurately, with which to depict our own dilemma of liberation? What shows up in work with individuals is that at some point, we can ask, "Where does this pattern come from?" and the response is usually as follows.

"It is mine now, but it has not always been mine; this is my mother's (father's, grandmother's) pattern."

"Why is it taken on by you?"

"I do it because I loved them and wanted things to be better."

"You take it on to make it better?"

"Yes."

At this point, or somewhere around this moment, a *metabasis* occurs, the neurochemistry shifts, and the pattern changes, often concluding.

One difficulty is in locating the held-energy systems, particularly when our chemistry reads the energy as invisible, non-existent, and forbidden. That its evocation may require the energetic presence of another, a person, within and/or without the mindbody, complicates our expectations for relationship with other people. No wonder we dwell in the shoals of "having faith," of interventionism, rather than in the depths of knowledge and discovery.

Christ Vision: Two Neurochemistries

Christ vision thus can carry the two neurochemistries with which we can encounter the energetic: its trusting, fluid and expansive mode, and the traumatic holding pattern, its initially life-saving rigidification of, for lack of a better term, Spirit. Which comes first is an intriguing, perhaps even amusing question, for as soon as the trust is vibrationally garnered, the "crucified" form emerges, impenetrably awaiting completion. We need to identify both phases in order to begin to experience freedom at the deepest cellular, molecular, atomic levels; only then will our systems self-balance.

Our Christ energy includes then both the clear and the held modes, in proximal, balanced, but ultimately dissatisfying oscillation. We are not content to witness Jesus merely die on the Cross, with no subsequent movement. Out of this understanding of our essential nature, our aspiration toward a Heaven is generated.

The dangers of clustering our superstitious focus around the rigidification of the recognition of Spirit in the figure of Jesus on the Cross could include a sadistic, narcissistic elaboration on the ending of life. Jesus himself as a person probably kindly disavowed such a formulation: "Forgive them, Father, for they know not what they do," as well as his persecutors' illusory dwelling upon narrative as essence, a commonplace problem over centuries.

The risk of not confronting the nature of the trauma mechanism and its narrative diversionary capacity is that we then may not witness the pattern in its full perpetration. We cannot allow the held energetic to resolve itself. This is a particular risk where we have religions whose lineages will not lead us to the point of dissolution of the oscillation between held- and non-held-energy Christ patterning.

Other individuals who have achieved high vibrational clarity, including Gautama Buddha, have died peacefully, even playfully accommodating their deaths in serenity. What is being celebrated when we celebrate the Christ in its Jesus narrative form, or better, when we address the energetic as *the* Christ, or for that matter, as I have done here, characterize energy as *the* energetic?

Though suffering is our door to resolution of trauma, by itself it is only midwife to our delivery. Suffering may be our reality, but is it the truth? Perhaps it would be preferable not to use the term Christ, with its heroic, paradoxical, hyperbolic vectors of perfection, and in implementation its susceptibility to the temptations of sentimentality and its sibling, cruelty. At least that has appeared to be a major part of Euro-American religious indoctrination. We should not be surprised when so-called Christian communities and individuals turn abusive, haplessly mistreating neighbors as themselves.

The image and life of Jesus have brought hope that narrative can be dropped and the energetic can be approached again, even in its most difficult, intractable forms. From the evidence of his sayings, certainly that was what interested him. If we see our modern times as increasing in violence and absurdity, could we see also that the patterns, the lineages of abuse are offering themselves up for resolution, in their most difficult forms?

We who carry them, such as the historically persecuted, may be within a hairsbreadth of resolving them, not just for now, but for millennia past. Each pogrom, each rape, each former-life abuse, each slavery, each addiction, each perpetration against self and other is an opportunity for healing, but the healing may not be complete until the lure of narrative which is founded upon trauma is understood and ignored.

APPENDIX: THERAPISTS AND ABUSE

Therapists and Abuse

The problem seems to be this: There have been violations of boundaries between clients and therapists, with damage to clients primarily being the realistic focus for concern. Also, therapists have encountered situations with clients wherein their sense of limits has been seriously challenged, particularly when clients have claimed abuse and the therapist denies abusing. Clients have been exploited sexually, throwing professions into consternation and at times confoundment with ethical concerns.

The most serious violations have occurred between vulnerable women clients and powerful male therapists, though the configurations have not been limited to that. There appears to be a breach of decorum and of the therapeutic norm, namely that clients and practitioners do not have sex together in the context of the therapeutic relationship.

In order to approach this delicate and explosive topic from a rock bottom place of what we can actually know about these situations, we may have to look at the therapeutic environment out of the context of current values and norms, in order to discover why our norms are being violated. If we want to conclude the violations, we may need to witness the energetic forces present, not just a confirmation of what we think is right and true.

The pain of taking this approach will seem obvious as you will note the oblique, at times arduous and convoluted prose which follows. My goal, however, is to recognize that dealing with these issues through language and law alone has not yet sufficed to bring a halt to the violations. Until we can approach them in an additional, alternate way, which I am proposing, we must stay within the linguistic norms, even though they may further entrap us and lead us to even greater harms. In no way am I condoning what has happened in the cases of therapeutic abuse, but I can see both parties as victims and as such am confounded when faced with issues of judgment.

Other kinds of abuse in therapy may be tolerated because they are less visible. Verbal, psychodynamic, relational, and energetic abuses may continue while the legal formulations of organ to organ interaction appear to protect the client or the therapist. Certainly this latter intervention may be a beginning, though it is only that. And to edge into the cataloguing and recognition of these more interior abuses leads us quickly into potentials for witchhunting, which in some cases has already occurred.

Yet a judge friend of mine movingly reports, how after hearing of the sexual abuses of one man upon all the members of his family, including his grandchildren, as judge my friend renders sentence on behalf of the family and of society, and I would add, of the man, by saying, "We will not tolerate this behavior. This must stop."

This legal beginning leads us into further legislation of trauma energetics, a possible origin of behavior which is incredibly difficult to appropriate through language, and which law has perhaps wisely chosen not to adjudicate. But we are heading to the impasses and limitations of language, as well as of behavior, whether we like it or not.

Consent to Orgasm in Therapy

No avenue to autonomous verbal consent to orgasmic sex within the therapeutic relationship has ever been found. One reason most often cited is that the client is in a power differential with the practitioner, which clouds his/her judgment by the probable transference of infantile feelings belonging to parental figures onto the therapist. In this event, the client/child cannot oppose the therapist/

parent's wishes. This important telling point can stop the so-identified sexual activity dead in its tracks. What the full abuse is which the victim feels or the perpetrator intends within the complex sexual encounter may be a more problematic question, and, I suspect, one which has not been fully documented by both (ir)responsible parties within such an encounter.

From another point of view, current understandings about what sex is have evolved under relational rubrics, so that the traditional formulations about sexual interaction are being challenged, including the challenge to *any* codification by participants or clinicians that objectifies the energetic reality of the interaction. Freud and his followers, including notably Reich, found themselves returning to an energetic understanding of personality and its original formulation in order to perceive the process by which the personality rigidifies and becomes objectified. Thus when we lose essential contact, abuse and contactlessness of so-called self and other result.

This means that even though we may envision sexual organs juxtaposed, between, say, client and therapist, we may be "witnessing" contactless sex, for some, a perhaps deeper violation than even interpenetration. We are thrown out of our traditional, simple moral assumptions about what is going on to an apperception of personal and spiritual crisis contained in the interaction. Though we know what has happened, we don't know what has been experienced.

To this end in the late twentieth century, sexuality has been seriously viewed not as a series of body/organ interactions, but more deeply as manifestation of various levels of energy interaction in the participants' mindbodies and in the interaction of mindbodies of the two partners. Here again, we are moving toward a yogic, meditational appreciation of what we have called our sexuality.

Obviously, various coupling patterns have been assessed (homosexual, intergenerational, etc.), and some people are still challenged by social, political and ethical concerns. At the cutting edge, however, many concerned people find the variations possible between partner couplings personally confounding, and in some cases, liberating. In other situations, the possibilities are experienced as frightening and destructive.

Viewed from this perspective, however, relating individuals reveal there is a darker sense of an interactional frontier, and it emerges in cases of violence and objectification of sexuality. In sexist, violent pornography, rape, abuse, etc., we see insecurities of personality as well as lineages of abuse which go back to childhood and before. These lead to patterns of abuse which people find legitimately threatening, both as acted on and acted upon, including in therapeutic settings.

It is against this background that the government is seeking to provide guidelines, albeit unsubtle ones, to protect the so-called innocent and the inexperienced.

Legal Guidelines

One major concern for "ethical" bodyworkers is that they somehow distinguish between their ethical non-orgasmic bodywork, and the massage parlor techniques which bring clients to orgasm. In order to develop and expand the levels of trust people have in touch, and in their bodies, it is crucial that those who want the former be not misled into the latter. Proposed laws support the objective that clients not be confronted with the possibility of violation of boundaries and expectations when they seek out ethical bodywork.

Amid this necessary correction and clarification of the therapeutic relationship, however, I see a hidden problem which I shall try to outline, one which emerges when we look at the subtler forms of therapeutic encounter, which may be obscured by current proposed legislation which attempts to protect client, and therapist, from violations.

Current legislation strategies include prohibition of touching, kissing, penetrating, etc. parts of the client's body which are sexually stimulating and "off-bounds." These can include breasts, buttocks, mouth, inner thighs, pelvic openings, etc. Exceptions are where the therapy-education lineages (for example, shiatsu, Rolfing, colon therapy, acupuncture, dentistry, jin shin jyutsu, polarity, etc.) include touch or penetration by fingers, needles, etc., as part of registered protocols, and are presumably not overtly, orgasmically sexual in intention.

The current crisis at the therapeutic level is one further aspect of some broad revolution of our relationship to sexual consciousness which has been proceeding in the West since before the *droite du seigneur*. Attitudes about appropriate and inappropriate modes of sexuality have been an issue for societies for the longest time. Current concerns date vividly from the Victorian period and come down through Freud and the neo-Freudians, into the current understandings of object relations theory and developmental psychology.

Developmental theorists propose that as bodies from the first we are linked with the world and ourselves by tactile experience. From a therapeutic perspective, the early experience of touch is part of what needs to be addressed in cases of dissociative experience. Thus in the context of a touch-deprived culture where by default sexuality has been linked to touch, the historical puritanical distrust of touch with its healing powers has been infrequently challenged. How can we estimate the cost to society and to individuals of this predisposition?

Again by default, there has been a societal abuse in its *nolo tangere* values which is currently being redressed slowly. The current differentiation between ethical massage and "prostitution" is designed to make touch respectable and desirable in the mind of the public. Don't people sorely need to find gentle and appropriate ways to enrich their private sensate experience in ways other than through objectified sexuality and violence? Those who do bodywork are trying to revaluate their positions in order that the clients feel safe in their presence so the work can be done.

Touch and Sexuality

To establish a point of entry into this minefield of feeling, action and psychology, we may have to ask, "What is the relationship between touch and sexuality?" While one answer may be, "It's obvious," a second consideration may reveal that we do not really know. If touch can be healing, can orgasmic sexuality also be considered healing, and under what conditions? And with whom?

If we start with, say, two people in a room, one way of looking at their interaction is to witness the space between them. How close are their bodies, what gestures do they make, and what are their responses to each other? The space between people, if there is one, can be bridged by touch, certainly, but it is defined more compellingly by energy. When approaching sexual intercourse, we are used to considering activities and feelings, which include touch, but I suspect our truest accounting of sexual potentiality does not so objectify, or better, densify, our incarnation.

One definition of sexuality involves that which is separate becoming joined. Because this energetic intuition is more confounding than it appears, the Freudian psychoanalytic lineage has declared that any touch is at base, sexual, and, with the exceptions of analysts who have jumped the fence, as it were, therefore must not be allowed by client or practitioner. Yet intuitively, energy is whole; it is not divided. When divided, it takes on the mantle of dissociation, as it were, with no chance for mutuality.

I wonder if there are not two contradicting positions here, one being that we can bring integrity to our actions, but not in the therapist's office, where our energy has been objectified into sexuality, specifically and universally by the prohibition to touch and to touch deeply.

Implicitly, for three or four generations of clients educated by contemporary therapists, and for centuries by religious organizations, we have been instructed that touch cannot be regulated with integrity. Beneath that is the obviation of our energetic reality which is more difficult to appropriate.

Self and Space

To understand their experience bridging the space between two bodies, most practitioners who do bodywork, including massage therapists, have adopted energetic strategies, including, for example, orgone, chi, Holy Spirit, prana, and kundalini. The idea of the self as a field center, a local, dense concentration of energy within a universal field, means that what heretofore was thought of as a discrete space between one body and the next is no longer understood that way.

Space is not empty space. It is an interface of energies which coalesce in the filtration or emphasis of skin and skin, these grossest lines of differentiation of bodies. This strategy enables the practitioner and client to find a way to set their experiences into balance, and into appropriate boundary definition. But in order to do that, most holistic practitioners see energies as influenceable across the space, and between bodies. They envision that the movement or influence of the energies can be intentional, as well as holistic.

If we see selves as whole or moving toward wholeness, then our definitions of what we practitioners are doing with those individuals has to transcend any particular moves or rhetorical protocol, though each practitioner evolves from particular lineages. Once one has learned more than one energetic strategy, the tendency is to adopt a more universal energetic strategy which encompasses, generalizes, or abstracts the insights of the particular lineages.

The hallmarks of most energy strategy synthesis can be perhaps best approached from the following positions:

The energy of the body is flowing, outward as well as inward-moving, relational, not objectified, not cut off in any one aspect of understanding or experience.

Wellness implies balance of these energies. Problems occur when there are "blocks" or blockages to this energy, which must be considered as universal and whole.

Consciousness may be seen as a codifier of these energies, reflecting and often partitioned from the whole, so that even consciousness has some features of dissociation to it, as with Freud's unconscious.

Even, or particularly, language involves this splitting off, dissociated quality. Tragically, in the attempt to describe energy which is the primary and usually hidden source of self-experience, even feelings, attitudes, and movement, the traditional gathering sites of self-experience, are secondary, and the language which describes them, tertiary. By describing, we risk promulgating that very dissociation.

The restoration of balance can occur when the practitioner invests intentionally some agency of intervention whose goal is to restore balance. This can include touch, pressure, acupuncture needles, whatever.

Energetic Paradigm of Sexuality

Our recent concern is that therapists have been violating the current boundary norms between therapist and client by having sex with clients. This begs the questions, "What is sex, and how is it to be limited or proscribed? In what setting is it allowed? Is sex healing?". Currently, society is revaluating this issue, and some attitudes have emerged.

A new paradigm is consolidating. Successful interpersonal interactions now reside within the concept of relational interactions, where we can focus, as it were, on the two people in the room. Buber's distinction between I-It and I-Thou interactions implies holistic interactions between two balanced mindbodies. As a result, there are a number of strategies to protect individuals from exploitation by therapists.

1. It is not the state's place to say what can go on between consenting adults. Yet what constitutes "consent" is problematic, and not just what appears at the surface.

2. Where violence and abuse occur in intimacies, social norms will be offered to victims who are caught in a web of sadomasochism in relationships, and legal protection will be offered. It is under this rubric, where the professional relationship between client and practitioner is fiduciary and one of trust, that the current laws are being revaluated.

3. Our ideal sexual "norm," perhaps fleetingly experienced, involves a sense of mutuality and appropriate pleasuring, where our sexual activities are negotiated throughout the interaction and can be terminated by either partner at any point in the process. Here with our consort, we can employ touch as an end in itself, never as a means.

4. Sexuality is not understood as a conjoining of organs, or body positions, or partners, all potentially varied, so much as a confluence of energies. Where there is dissociation, our erotic energies objectify—into sexuality and further into ritualized objectified sexuality. Our relationship will not be Buber's I-Thou, but rather I-It. Higher levels of vibrational interaction suggest forms of sexuality not usually condoned or developed by traditional authorities.

5. When, under the pressure of traumatic processing, our energy systems fractionate, they objectify, into language as well as within the internal experience of individuals. It is this fractionation which theorists see as damaging, resulting in alienation and violence, between people and peoples.

6. Every process of legal limit-setting involves the risk that our energies will be fractionated further, substituting a retraumatization, as it were, rather than a holistic discovery of our unity of self and our unity of self with another. The spiritual and social importance of this goal cannot be underestimated. The failures of fractionated consciousness, apparently accelerating in the twentieth century, are manifold.

7. The negotiation of the space between individuals is critical to our discussion of sexuality, for it is here that the acts which start as energetic become incarnated into the material and physical world, specifically the mindbody. Our interactions do not have to be those of bumper cars.

8. How we let another mindbody into our general energy field, or return the energy outward toward another person, becomes the dance of courtship and experience, intention and surrender of intention, one which legislators exclusively delineate at our peril. While some people are intimidated by laws opposing violations of integrity to themselves and others, many, increasingly, are not, nor do they understand or experience the wholeness which integrity implies. Setting down laws does not stop our traumata from being violationally expressed.

9. Past legislation attempting to control sexuality, including homosexuality or women's sexuality, often has damaged individuals who have then had to seek political redress, at perilous cost to themselves and others. The resultant damage to persons and to personality by church and state has been overt, covert, political, and appalling.

10. The social requirements and guidelines for individual safety must be established within a framework whose goal is to allow people to find their balance, though this is impossible to regulate externally and even under the greatest care and experience, is subject to huge misunderstandings, at the very least.

11. With this in mind, holistic practitioners seek to reduce the excesses rendered by traditional medicine, which often has objectified relationships and fractionated our mindbody experience, only to be frustrated by reversion to old, self-destructive sexual mores.

12. The self itself is an objectified concept, and as a strategy for delineation of what occurs between people has its risks.

13. Silence. In response to our rhetoric about sexuality and the actual practices and experiences which people have in this realm, words often provide sad, and inadequate commentary.

14. Where our energy is appropriately whole and resonant with vibrational trust, we may encounter traumatic dissociation, which engenders our focusing upon the "source" of our center. Instead of energy, we conceive the source of our actions as drive to power, to sexuality, to whatever can be objectified. Yet if self is a way of identifying a density within a wider surround, it becomes devilishly difficult to negotiate our way through a shared energy field and to take responsibility as a practitioner as well as as a client, particularly if the client has trauma interfering with awareness. No matter how whole our energy field is, it is hard to see it as from the outside, or from the inside, hence the concerns among practitioners about projection and transference, which are merely guidelines for our orientation through these energy fields.

Sexual Energetics

In the reductionist abstractions which have coalesced in theory and now, primarily, in the alternative health and growth culture, viewing sexual interactions from an energetic point of view clarifies the nature of abuse in an attempt to stop it and to restore balance and respect to the participants in intercourse of all kinds. Feminist and men's liberationist writing, sex education texts, and religious denominational teachings, to name the most prominent voices in this dialogue, all proclaim the goal of healthy relationship to the body, including appropriate sexuality. Sectarian differences arise in the determination of what that goal means and how it is manifest.

When we see the violence between sexes and within personality as a function not of forces for divisiveness but of divisions which are striving to be brought together, important questions become visible: "What are the sections of personality to be brought together, and how did they originally arise as sections?" To get to the basis of a viewpoint transcending any one particular manifestation within the personality or between personalities, clinical and theoretical lineages have adopted with increasing complexity an energetic view of our mindbody. This perspective postulates various impasses preventing active, generous, and loving flow of energy throughout our mindbody and "outward" toward others.

Within that context, the Freudian libido strategy, the Reichian orgone, the Chinese chi and qigong, the Indian kundalini and prana, the Christian Holy Spirit, all seek resolution of cognitive impasses with the concept of energy. For this reason, it is at this interface between the cognitive and the energetic that any legal intervention faces its greatest challenge.

A developmental sequence of personality suggests that because of experiences both within and without individual mindbodies, we come to see ourselves in rigid as well as energetically fluid ways, with our actual behavior often contradictorily, or paradoxically juxtaposed to our "conscious" view of self. Socially, our modern concepts of relationship appear still rigidly archaic, and in flux. For example, gender roles are being revaluated under this rubric with even the tiniest changes causing upheavals.

One goal amid all this change is that our energy become whole, that we do not split mind from body, sexuality from love, special, shall we say eroticized, parts of the body from other parts. A major goal in current therapy is that when we review early childhood when presumably the false and true differentiations of adulthood, gained through trauma and experience, are not manifest, we can respond with openness and trust.

Viewing Wholeness

Various adult and differentiated centers from which to view this wholeness are significant, and traditionally include power, money, sex, love, and spirit. We can start at one of these fractional viewing points and work in and through each to a sense of wholeness. When viewed from any one of these positions, let us say the sexual, we may simplify and say, "All human experience is based upon our sexual nature. Beneath everything is sex," a position which attempts to serve a vision of wholeness from a split-off, reductionist point of view.

To say that everything can be simplified to economics, or to affirm, "Power is what determines our actions," or "Everything can be resolved into the spiritual," reflects a similar linguistic and ideational strategy, simultaneously recognizing our need for wholeness, but observing it from a place of linguistic, conceptual division.

The reason these strategies are important is that when the law is evolving, lawyers and politicians are also attempting a similar strategy, this time from a legal point of view, trying to establish through language and ideation some balance, called justice, in the face of energetic wholeness. Yet the energetic, sexual-energetic, in this case, is essentially not divided, and any attempt to ignore this fact dooms the law's implementation to manipulation and abuse, either by its employment or its lack of employment.

When we enter the office of a therapist or bodyworker, we intend to rework safely some of the patterns which were laid down in early childhood, when boundary diffusion is a challenge in life. Getting to a more holistic and integrated experience of ourselves means returning to non-verbal, tactile exchanges which bodywork now offers. Therefore, it is the negotiation of these boundaries which body and verbal work combined now present as a reachable synthesis.

The movement between verbal—more developed and abstract, but also more split-off—and non-verbal energetic communication offers hope to clients who heretofore have been able to rely only on the verbal interactions for redefinition and reworking of old trauma, deprivations, etc. Thus, legally dividing therapy into two distinct segments, verbal and body work, as reportedly is currently the case in one western state, arbitrarily reinforces the destructive, retraumatizing division in our society and culture currently manifest in these delicate areas of cutting-edge relationality where touch and verbal expression interface. Clients are haplessly thrown into a room with a practitioner who is also inexperienced in the shared energetic reality of the sexual, spiritual, and power matrices of their interaction. And in their wounded energetic, they seek healing by finding a sexual narrative.

Energy and Sexual Abuse

Operating with a wounded, traumatized, and dissociated model of self and other, the practitioner is surprised to find him/herself "seduced" into the energetic areas of boundary fusion and delineation which he/she then perceives in a dissociated way as sexual. He/she acts upon them, honoring these sensations as being honest, or real, or beyond conscious, *i.e.*, dissociated, control. Or he/she acts upon them in part because they are forbidden or because he/she is inexperienced, or because he/she is tired of transferential perpetration through non-touch. He/she perpetrates in personal areas where the culture has concealed or monolithically and superficially examined and labelled experience. Where there are multiplicities of levels of interaction, society, including the practitioner's professional supervisors, only offer one.

The original abuse has set off the trauma mechanism, which, like the household electrical circuit breaker, is a neurochemical response which naturally immobilizes and protects the neurochemical system of personality from complete burnout, annihilation, and destruction. The client has been left with fractionated, commemorative held-energy systems which then continue to interfere in the natural flow of outward-moving energy which continues to flow, sometimes filtered and channelled through these systems. This is the harvest of abuse.

Like the client's, the practitioner's traumata are always pushing to the front of the line in his/her personality to get appropriately completed. The fragile energy at the center of being which has been protectively immobilized by our mindbody system in order to survive now demands appropriate, full, and safe completion of the gesture which initially has been truncated by the traumatic process. In the context of trust, one-way and mutual between practitioner and client, the second shoes of trauma are (removed and) dropped.

It might be argued that all violations between therapist and client currently under examination in the press are the effect of at least two held-energy systems bumping haplessly against each other. In each the dissociated, held energy tries to become whole and moving again, hence in these cases, the move toward so-called sexual activity. These "violations" spring from the attempt to redress imbalances, implicitly based upon black, held energy within both people, on both sides of client-practitioner fences.

The nature of dissociation, however, makes it difficult to weed out what is good from what is split-off within both partners. Hence a deeper model of relationality has to be devised than one which merely retreats to an object relations level of differentiation between self and other, already dangerously objectified and retraumatizing. Legal jargon tends to support non-energetic views of personality. For example, it does not recognize the reality of energy work, hence it may be a curiously inappropriate tool to delineate fully this problem.

Because our most severe levels of disturbance, the original confusions or trauma patterns, are laid down probably before we can speak, not to touch, nor to offer touch, can be as abusive as currently touching is strategized by mainstream non-touching therapists. It can no longer be easily accepted that the practitioner/therapist is not retraumatizing the client if he/she refrains from touch. Not touching is no longer *a priori* safe nor a sign of non-abusive treatment just because it advances under the no-orgasm flag.

It is also true that touching even by responsible clients and practitioners does not miraculously promise relief from the confounding boundary issues in extreme cases of trauma, such as those presented by the therapeutically "difficult" so-called "borderline" clients, now more appropriately seen as suffering from post-traumatic stress. The energetic distortions of held-energy systems out of which behavioral and psychological abuses arise make us all vulnerable to pattern perpetration which even the narrative forms of touch may not resolve.

The client/practitioner relationship must expand toward clarification of the developmental movement from touch to words, from touch to non-touch, from boundary fusion-diffusion to boundary differentiation. This requires the imaginative participation of both practitioner and client on a more equal, relational footing than has been heretofore generally ascribed in therapeutic encounters, particularly in cases of severe trauma.

Thus any law which seeks to generally protect the client, especially the abused client, in its objectification of sexuality into restricted body parts and movements, may not deal with the primary energetic reality from which the confusion arises and to which it must return if the original held-energy system is to be dissolved. In the service of getting clarity about what practitioner/therapists are supposed not to do, such law may be retraumatizing.

The Future Place for Law in Therapeutic Lineages

Where does this vision leave us? Are we to have no legal guidelines? Certainly the educational force of the law is promulgating changes in the ways therapists are interacting with their clients. Perhaps some perpetrations are being stalled, though in the mindbodies of the perpetrators, probably not resolved by "abstinence" any more than by perpetration.

Positively, the new guidelines are giving people a focal point for their expectations about therapy, a deepening of their understanding of the radical violations which have occurred, as well as of the more subtle, and perhaps more pernicious violations implicit in the current traditional therapeutic paradigms which are accepted as safe. If the law takes us this far, more power to it.

Yet I wonder whether some of this educational force of law holds significant risks for the development of therapeutic encounters beyond our current, often ineffective treatment hiatus. Under inquisitional pressures, the safest way is to revert to the status quo (C.Y.A.) which is comfortable, self-selected among like-personalitied therapeutic lineages, and because not examined, often radically perpetrative.

When we run into exceptional situations as have happened recently, we can glimpse how precarious the therapeutic lineage, for radicals and conservatives alike, actually is. Adventuresome, imperfect, traumatically bound therapists are supervised by top, establishment people in volatile cases which turn awry, even mortal. Under public pressure, top people then appear to abandon ship, and implement the status quo. A section of the lineage is torn up, and we see how superficial our orthodox, "professional" understanding has been.

GLOSSARY

aura the electromagnetic and sometimes subtle energy surrounds of the mindbody which suffuse, penetrate, and densify into chemistry and tissue.

bardo a strategy describing states and processes beyond death.

bottoming out a therapeutic strategy suggesting we must psychologically touch the bottom of the pool before we can push up to the surface again.

clear the apparent highest vibration state, beyond color, beyond golden, wherein the balance of the personality has no holding in it. Short of that we are in color, in denser vibration.

dissociation a much-used term variously describing altered states of chemistry and personality not thought usual, involving some concept of trauma or separation from true, centered being.

encapsulation a sense of traumatically held aspects of personality with boundaries which do not allow movement or information through them. In personality, it conveys bound energy, either at the edge of the so-called personality as it interfaces with other personality fields, or as islands within the personality.

energy that sense of being which vitalizes us. Subtle energy is beyond regularly recordable electromagnetic waves, and pertains to incarnation strategy *held-energy system* The offspring of the trauma mechanism. It is the remainder of what does not get resolved by a traumatic experience after the organism is restored to mobility. It registers as black in our internal scan, and controls or appears to control further density levels such as movement in the brain, muscles, and neurophysiological structures.

incarnation If we use a mind/body strategy, at some point we can view experience as spirit (Spirit) progressively densifying into our mortal, final flesh. If we want to perceive the Godhead, or get as close as we can get to whatever that is, we might focus upon that which is prior to the smallest perceivable, recordable phenomenon. We ask what is it that is the causal point of origin of that, say quark. The response is Spirit, or God. In this sense incarnation might show the following "descent": God/Spirit, sub-atomic elements/energy, atoms, neurochemistry, electromagnetic field, neurochemistry/molecules, cells, tissue, organs, structure. Parallel to these physical densities can be included fundamentalist convictions, emotions, ideas, body images, personality traits, personality, though these not in any special order. Incarnation insight suggests the Godhead can be perceived at any point in experience, not just the smallest reducible one.

intention directives or thought patterns which sense as if ego is moving the inner furniture where it wants.

narrative everything which is not spirit. Narrative can be the story of our life, personality, a disease process, a psychological explanation of something, an insight, our perceptions of our bodies, etc. When we are not in narrative, we are in the energetic, particularly confronting our held-energy systems, which, because of their neurochemical difficulty, appear to propel brain into narrative.

neurochemistry our molecular, electromagnetic, enzymatic being; our molecules, organelles and organismic nature viewed as chemistry.

pattern a sequence which reveals the structure of an invisible held-energy system. This can be manifest at any level—psychodynamic, cellular, relational, physical, etc. I also use the term pattern to describe this underlying structure, which is the land's end viewing promontory interfacing with subtle energy, the spirit, and mystery.

pre-windshield chaos the moment of profound disequilibrium prior to hitting the windshield, which sets off the trauma mechanism, with its objectifying rigidifications designed to preserve the integrity of the mind-body. In these moments our mindbody reverts to early core or spindle traumata solutions, the ones which got us through before.

titrating diluting, approaching the toxicities of held-energy systems slowly, so we do not get overwhelmed by the information and thus cannot see what the process is.

tragictatus most tragic, wherein the full cycle of the tragic is played out, is allowed to move from impaction into full cellular openness. We are not left with dead-end despair, but are shown how balance is restored out of that.

trauma mechanism the neurochemistry which suspends the life force and turns our mindbody into a rigidification to preserve its integrity. It produces held-energy systems which are a residue of this mechanism.

trust reciprocal vibratory interface, of one mindbody field with another, vibrating openly in homeostasis. I intuit that the deepest levels of trust do not have trauma or held energy within them.

vibration movement, apperceivable in sound, color, time. One aspect of life.

IDIOSYNCRATIC BIBLIOGRAPHY

Almaas, A.H. *Essence, The Diamond Approach to Inner Realization*. Samuel Weiser Inc., York Beach, Maine, 1988.

Arendt, Hannah. *The Origins of Totalitarianism, Parts One, Two, Three*. Harvest Book 131, 132, 133, Harcourt Brace & World, New York, 1968.

Arendt, Hannah. *Between Past and Future, Eight Exercises in Political Thought*. Viking Press, New York, 1968.

Austen, Jane. *Lady Susan, The Watsons, Sanditon*. editor Margaret Drabble, Penguin Books, 1975.

Austen, Jane. *The Complete Novels of Jane Austen*..The Modern Library, New York, 1933.

Bataille, Georges. *Death and Sensuality, A Study of Eroticism and the Taboo*. Walker and Company, New York, 1962.

Blake, William. *Poetical Works of William Blake*. Edited with Introduction by John Sampson, New York, Oxford University Press, 1913.

Bion, Wilfred R.. *Seven Servants, Four Works*. Jason Aronson, Inc. New York, NY, 1977.

Brennan, Barbara Ann. *Hands of Light, A Guide to Healing Through the Human Energy Field*. Bantam Books, New York, 1988.

Buber, Martin. *I and Thou*. Scribners, New York, 1970.

Cecil, David. *A Portrait of Jane Austen*. Hill and Wang, New York, 1978.

Coleridge, Samuel Taylor. *Coleridge Selected Poetry & Prose*. Edited by Stephen Potter. Nonesuch Press, London, 1962.

Dürckheim, Karlfried Graf. Hara, The Vital Centre of Man. Translated from the German by Sylvia-Monica von Kospoth, In collaboration with Estelle R. Healy. Mandala (an Imprint of Harper Collins), London 1988.

Funahashi, Shintaro, Bruce, Charles J., and Goldman-Rakic, Patricia S., "Mnemonic Coding of Visual Space in the Monkey's Dorsolateral Prefrontal Cortex," Journal of Neurophysiology, Vol 61, No. 2, February 1989, pp 331-349.

Goldman, Patricia S. "Neuronal Plasticity in Primate Telencephalon: Anomalous Projections Induced by Prenatal Removal of Frontal Cortex," Science, Vol. 202, 17 November 1978, pp 768-770.

Hillman, James. "Oedipus Revisited," *Oedipus Variations*. Spring Publications Inc., Dallas, Texas, 1991.

Hobbes, Thomas. *Leviathan*. Introduction by A.D. Lindsay, Everyman's Library, E.P. Dutton Co. Inc. N.Y. 1950.

Jones, John. *On Aristotle and Greek Tragedy*. Chatto & Windus, London, 1962.

Leavis, Q.D. "A Critical Theory of Jane Austen's Writing (II): 'Lady Susan' Into 'Mansfield Park'," Scrutiny, Vol X, No. 2, October, 1941, pp 114-142.

Leavis, Q.D. "A Critical Theory of Jane Austen's Writing (II): 'Lady Susan' Into 'Mansfield Park' (ii)," Scrutiny, Vol X, No. 3, January, 1942, pp 272-294.

Leavis, Q.D. "A Critical Theory of Jane Austen's Writing," Scrutiny, Vol X, No. 1, June 1941, pp 61-87.

Levine, Peter. *Encountering the Tiger: How the Body Heals Trauma*. Prepublication Manuscript, 1991.

Mack, Burton L. *The Lost Gospel, The Book of Q & Christian Origins*. Harper, San Francisco, 1993.

McGuire, Philip K., Bates, Julianna F., Goldman-Rakic, and Patricia S. "Interhemispheric Integration: I. Symmetry and Convergence of the Corticocortical Connections of the Left and the Right Principal Sulcus (PS) and the Left and the Right Supplementary Motor Area (SMA) in the Rhesus Monkey," Cerebral Cortex, Sept/Oct 1991; 1:390-407; 1047-3211/91.

McGuire, Philip K., Bates, Julianna F., and Goldman-Rakic, Patricia S. "Interhemispheric Integration: II. Symmetry and Convergence of the Corticostriatal Projections of the Left and the Right Principal Sulcus (PS) and the Left and the Right Supplementary Motor Area (SMA) in the Rhesus Monkey," Cerebral Cortex, Sept/Oct 1991; 1:408-417; 1047-3211/91.

McKeon, Richard, ed. *The Basic Works of Aristotle*. Random House, New York, 1941.

Plato. *The Republic and Other Works*. Translated by B. Jowett. Anchor Books, New York, 1973.

Poulet, Georges. *Studies in Human Time*. Translated by Elliot Coleman, The Johns Hopkins Press, Baltimore and London, 1956.

Raphael, Chester M. "DOR Sickness—A Review of Reich's Findings," CORE (Cosmic Orgone Engineering) Vol. VII, Nos 1-2; March 1955, Orgone Institute Press, Rangeley Maine, pp. 20-28.

Reich, Wilhelm, with Robert A. McCullough. "Melanor, Orite, Brownite and Orene," CORE (Cosmic Orgone Engineering) Vol. VII, Nos 1-2; March 1955, Orgone Institute Press, Rangeley Maine, pp. 29-39.

Reich, Wilhelm. *Contact With Space. Oranur, Second Report, 1951-1956, OROP Desert Ea, 1954-1955*, Core Pilot Press, New York 1957, [United States Court of Appeals For the First Circuit, No 5160, Record Appendix to Briefs For Appellants Vol V. Secret and Suppressed Evidence OROP Desert Ea 1954-1955 "Wilhelm Reich et. at., Defendants- Appellants V. United States of America, Appeller"].

Reich, Wilhelm. "The Blackening Rocks," Orgone Energy Bulletin, Vol. V, Nos 1-2; March, 1953, Orgone Institute Press, Rangeley, Maine, pp. 28-59.

Reich, Wilhelm. "The Oranur Experiment, First Report (1947-1951)," Orgone Energy Bulletin, Vol. 3, Nos 4; October, 1951, Orgone Institute Press, Rangeley, Maine, pp. 185-344.

Sharaf, Myron. *Fury on Earth, A Biography of Wilhelm Reich*, St. Martin's Press/Marek, New York, 1983.

Skinner, B.F., "Superstition in the Pigeon," Journal of Experimental Psychology, Vol. 38, 1948, American Psychological Association, Washington, D.C., pp. 168-172.

Steinberg, Leo. *The Sexuality of Christ in Renaissance Art and Modern Oblivion.* Pantheon/October Book, New York, 1983.

Thakar, Vimala. *The Eloquence of Living.* New World Library, San Raphael, California, 1989.

INDEX

Aeschylus 15, 19, 75
    Agamemnon 89
    Eumenides 90
    Oresteia 90
Almaas, A.H. 121, 361
Aquinas, St. Thomas 152, 293
Arendt, Hannah 26, 361
Aristotle ... 8, 12, 13, 15, 18, 22, 23,
        28, 29, 81, 90, 362, 363
    Cresphontes 15
    Poetics 8, 9
Austen, Jane . 20, 21, 23, 24, 34, 44,
              104, 361
    Emma 20-25
    Harriet 21-23
    Leavis, Queenie 362
    Mansfield Park 20
    Mr. Knightley 21, 22
    Northanger Abbey 20
    Persuasion 21, 23
    Pride and Prejudice 20
    Sanditon 21, 23, 361
    Sense and Sensibility 20
Bataille, Georges 26, 361
Bergson, Henri 59
Biblical references, figures
    Abraham 90, 306, 307
    Adam 295, 297
    burning bush 305, 316
    Eve 295, 297
    Genesis 293-296, 298, 299,
        305, 308, 309, 320, 323
    Isaac 90, 306, 307
    Jerusalem 292
    Jesus . 15, 74, 90, 91, 124, 125,
  144, 224, 303, 304, 306-308, 310-
  312, 315-318, 320, 330-333, 335,
            337, 338
    Lucifer 28
    Moses .. 88, 305, 306, 321, 324
    St. Paul 300
    Ten Commandments .. 305, 316
Blake, William ... 93, 94, 149, 292,
              361
Buber, Martin 361
clients, named
    Andrew 67-70
    Doris 70
    Eleanor 326
    Elise 64
    Erica 62, 63
    Frieda 154-156
    Grace 51, 166, 167
    Harry 72
Coleridge, Samuel T. 82, 362
Conrad, Joseph 20
Darwin, Charles 294
Descartes, René 104
energetic color
    beige 116
    black . 3, 68, 70, 72, 83-85, 88-
  90, 92, 97, 100, 101, 104-119,
  121-123, 132, 133, 136, 142, 151, 155,
  156, 159-162, 166, 171, 172, 175, 177,
  179, 181, 184, 187, 191-193, 195,
  197-199, 203, 208, 210, 214, 216, 217,
  219, 227, 228, 230, 244, 245, 247-254,
  256, 257, 263-267, 274, 275, 278-280,
  282-284, 287, 296, 298, 299, 302, 325,
  331, 333, 353, 358
    blue .. 104, 118, 143, 212, 215,
          226, 244, 255

brown 100, 111, 116, 127,
142, 161, 198, 199, 253-256, 288
gold 118, 119
gray 48, 84, 114-116, 118,
142, 169-171, 204, 205, 211, 212
green ... 3, 117, 118, 166, 180,
181, 186, 187, 189-191, 193-195,
244, 253, 255, 259, 281
orange 115, 116
pink 117
purple 116, 117, 119, 191,
193
red . 3, 117, 121, 122, 128, 183,
191-193, 211, 214, 215, 217, 250
silver 48, 89, 115
tan 111, 116
white 12, 46, 48, 109-112,
114-117, 122, 128, 142, 170, 171,
191, 247, 258, 259
yellow 100, 116-118
energetic concepts
chakra ... 5, 83, 126, 193, 223,
291
interface .. 1, 12, 33, 44, 62, 82,
95, 99, 100, 117, 119, 124, 128,
136, 138, 147, 151, 162, 180, 192,
208, 221, 225, 236, 263, 277, 301, 304,
326, 329, 345, 350, 351, 359
juxtaposition 51, 115, 124,
277
skew............ 1, 123, 125
torque 123, 133, 162
vector 19, 61, 67, 121-125,
128, 136, 190, 215, 232, 255, 257,
266, 297, 299
vibration 67, 73, 76, 83, 84,
98, 111, 118, 119, 125, 128, 150,
152, 166, 191, 254, 263, 298, 315,
357, 359
energetic forms 185
amoeboid 1, 124
cave 81
cross .. 123-125, 136, 192, 209,
313, 319, 333-335, 337
crumbling 127
cuboid 120
diamond 85, 121, 140, 157,
361

edge . 2, 21, 66, 75, 78, 85, 165,
173, 340, 341, 351, 357
faceted jewel 121
flat 30, 45, 127, 177
funnel 126
line ... 20, 50, 74, 99, 103, 115,
117, 119, 121, 123, 127, 131, 136,
140, 166, 167, 214, 227, 231, 255, 264,
267, 298, 318, 352
melting 106, 122
mirror ... 16, 25, 115, 123, 317
peeling 127, 188, 266
plane 127
plastic 48, 127-129, 142
rectangle 248
right angle 124, 255, 334
solid .. 148, 162, 177, 187, 263,
335
spinning 126
square 120, 249
surface 17, 41, 44, 85, 100,
115, 121, 122, 126, 127, 179, 181-
188, 194, 205, 232, 251, 254, 346,
357
triangle 33
tube 122, 127
tunnel 127, 261
void 84, 119, 152, 299
vortex 126, 166, 225, 226,
309
whirlpool 223
energetic surfaces
corrugated 106, 122
glossy 115, 122, 194
matte 85, 115, 122, 172
mirror ... 16, 25, 115, 123, 317
rough 106, 122, 172
smooth 106, 122
energy, names of ... 3, 59-61, 64, 67,
76, 82, 105, 108, 206, 312, 329-
332, 335, 336, 345, 350, 363
chi 47, 59, 345, 350
elan vitale 59
eros ... 33, 63, 64, 68, 94, 160,
308, 309, 324
Holy Spirit .. 59, 317, 331, 345,
350

kundalini ... 59, 142, 299, 345, 350
libido 59, 88, 350
life force . 55, 59-61, 63, 65, 68, 77, 84, 90, 105, 150, 253, 299, 359
prana 59, 345, 350
qigong 350
spirit ... 12, 14, 18, 39, 42, 52, 59, 61, 67, 69, 74, 86, 87, 166, 168, 291, 294, 303, 305, 306, 310, 311, 317, 331, 336, 337, 345, 350, 358, 359
subtle energy ... 29, 44, 81, 82, 85, 91, 119, 149, 160, 162, 192, 223, 310, 357, 359
Equus 132
Euripides 15
Hahnemann, Samuel 59
Hegel, G.W.F............. 93, 292
Hobbes, Thomas 20, 159, 362
Homer
Odysseus 89, 91, 142
Odyssey 91, 92, 254
Penelope 89, 91
Sirens 91
Telemachus 89, 91, 142
Hunt, Valerie 5, 210, 310
Ibsen, Henrik 20
Kafka, Franz 80, 172
Karesh, David 331
Luther, Martin 322, 323
Malcolm X 108, 110
Marx, Karl 292
Marxism 292
Merope 15, 22, 90
Miller, Arthur 19
Plato...................... 363
Poulet, Georges 48, 363
psychological terms .. 10, 11, 14, 16, 17, 19, 22, 23, 25, 26, 28, 30, 31, 38, 39, 43, 44, 79, 80, 147, 160, 269, 271, 292, 298, 299, 302, 304, 318, 349
release 34, 66, 77, 91, 255, 292, 299
superstitious pigeon 107
transference .. 30, 34, 147, 268, 269, 271, 272, 286, 302, 340, 349
Racine, Jean Baptiste 19

Rashomon 60
religious groups ... 14, 51, 125, 144, 280, 299, 307-309, 311, 312, 316-320, 323, 332, 338, 350, 362
Buddhist ... 150, 317, 319, 335
Catholic .. 317, 318, 322, 323, 325
Jew ... 305, 315-317, 320, 322, 324, 331
Protestant 35, 49, 51, 321, 322, 324, 325
Rolfing ... 43, 52-54, 62, 63, 67, 145, 165, 270, 342
connective tissue 52-54
Rolf, Ida 52-54
Rolfee 53, 54
Rolfer 43, 53, 54, 270
Rousseau, Jean Jacques
Rousseau 292
Second Council of Constantinople 318
Sens, Timothy .... ix, 334
Shakespeare, William 15
Shaw, G.B. 20, 59
Snow White 12, 46
Sophocles.............. iv, 15, 19
Creon 92
Oedipus . iv, 16, 19, 28, 92, 93, 113, 151, 241, 362
Oedipus at Colonus ... 92, 114, 151, 241
Oedipus Rex 16, 28, 113
spiritual concepts . 60, 102, 330, 334, 335
Buddha 74, 118, 156, 232, 304, 310, 317, 337
Christ .. 64, 97, 110, 118, 144, 156, 232, 311, 315, 316, 320, 329-337, 364
Covenant ... 154, 299, 302-306, 309, 311, 315-317, 321, 325, 332
Crucifixion 124, 307, 310, 312, 332-335
determinism 9, 49, 97, 137
evil 107, 298-300, 323
free will 137
Garden of Eden .. 113, 295, 321
Gautama Buddha 74, 337

Heaven 52, 93, 292, 337
incarnate . . 14, 29, 67, 85, 149,
          259, 299, 303, 331
incarnation . . 52, 67, 74, 76, 86,
87, 124, 140, 162, 165, 277, 296,
305, 306, 319, 320, 344, 357, 358
innocence 26, 94, 95, 97
innocence and experience . . 94,
          95, 97
Life After Death 51, 318
Messiah . . . 301, 303, 304, 310-
          312, 332, 333, 335
Nirvana 292, 319
Original Sin 112, 296, 297,
          318, 323
political religion 291, 305,
          316, 319
reincarnation . . 49-52, 317, 318
Resurrection 90, 306, 318,
          332, 333, 335
right action . . 29, 71, 81, 82, 99,
          240
salvation . . . 300, 302, 310, 317,
          319
Satan 107, 299, 300
Savior . 300-304, 310, 312, 332,
          333, 335
Second Coming . 313, 318, 324
Tao 59, 119
The Cross . . 123-125, 313, 333-
          335, 337
structural integration 52, 53
Suddenly, Last Summer 132
symbolist 135
Thakar, Vimala . . . . ix, 1, 55, 82, 97,
          152, 364
therapies . . 24, 29, 30, 35, 37, 41, 42,
44, 45, 47, 53, 85, 86, 114, 137,
138, 142, 154, 157, 343, 346
bioenergetic 3, 44, 45, 220
Jin Shin 343
psychodrama 42, 85
reflexology 45
Reiki 59, 86, 145
therapists
Bergler, Edmund 46
Bion, Wilfred 98, 361

Brennan, Barbara Ann 126,
          361
Dillenger, George ix
Freud, Sigmund . . 9, 14, 16, 29,
35, 61, 66, 86-88, 90, 103, 114,
148, 174, 312, 341, 343
Heppe, Wilhelm . . . ix, 118, 119
Hochwender, Mark . . . . ix, 151
Jung, C. G. 35
Keene, Rosemary . . . . ix, 45
. . . Levine, Peter . . . ix,1-4, 55, 57,
61, 67, 77, 84, 133, 154, 202,
          362
Lowen, Alexander 42, 272
Moreno, J.L. 42
Pierrakos, John . . . . ix, 3, 4, 42
Reich, Wilhelm . 42, 43, 61, 83,
88, 108, 148, 149, 333, 341, 363
Sharaf, Myron . . ix, 42, 83, 88,
          108, 363
Tiffen, Gregge . . . . ix, 47, 50-52
tragic theory, concepts
anagnōrisis . . . 21, 55, 121, 296
character . . . 14, 16, 19, 23, 29,
          43, 44, 59, 148
dramatis personae 11, 65
fear 7, 28, 36, 55, 88, 126,
          132, 155, 171, 261, 262
hamartia 23
hero . . 8-10, 12, 14, 19, 28, 88,
          320, 332
imitation . . . 13, 29, 30, 75, 82,
          100, 115, 298, 332
katharsis 29
metabasis . . . 18, 19, 55, 90, 91,
          336
mimēsis . 29, 81, 331, 332, 334
muthos 8, 16, 295, 333
peripeteia 8, 19, 55
pity 28
plot . 12, 16, 19, 28, 29, 85, 89,
          92, 113, 117
praxis 16, 18, 29
scapegoat 8, 14, 15, 28
serious action . . . 13, 18-20, 23,
          29, 30, 65, 74, 75, 81, 166
stasis 15, 44, 55, 63, 158

tragedy . 6, 8-16, 18-22, 25-28, 30, 31, 44, 55, 81, 90, 332, 362
tragic ... 6, 8-12, 14, 15, 18, 19, 21-23, 25-31, 55, 65, 67, 75, 81, 88, 90, 91, 110, 112, 166, 305-307, 316, 332, 359
tragictatus .. 15, 18, 22, 23, 26, 90, 359
trauma energetic strategies ... iv, 1-6, 11-14, 16, 17, 19, 21, 22, 24-26, 28-30, 42-47, 49, 52-55, 57, 64-71, 73-95, 98-100, 102, 104-106, 108-112, 115-120, 122-129, 132-136, 138-141, 144-151, 154-157, 160-162, 166, 167, 171, 173, 174, 176-178, 181, 185, 192, 195, 198, 203, 205-208, 210, 212, 214, 216-221, 223-225, 227, 229, 230, 236, 239, 241, 253-255, 262, 263, 266, 269, 271, 272, 277, 285-287, 291, 296-310, 316-318, 320, 321, 323, 325, 327, 330-341, 344-346, 348-354, 357-359
action ... 13, 14, 16, 18-20, 23, 26, 29, 30, 41, 65, 71, 74, 75, 81, 82, 92, 99, 142, 166, 240, 295, 298, 325, 334, 344
activity . 13, 18, 20, 23, 30, 33, 59, 65, 70, 91, 92, 94, 105, 299, 320, 341, 353
alchemical 150
bottoming out .. 15, 17, 22, 90, 307, 357
breath 137, 138, 228, 326
change 7, 18-20, 26, 54, 55, 59, 62, 71, 72, 75, 78, 81, 85, 90-92, 98, 102, 116-118, 126, 131-133, 140, 141, 143, 150, 154-157, 160, 166, 167, 182, 214, 215, 219, 220, 224, 228, 237, 244, 248, 250, 255, 263, 264, 270, 275, 300, 350
clear 38, 42, 43, 50, 55, 66, 74, 92, 93, 95, 97, 104, 107, 111, 119-121, 124, 134, 136, 137, 142, 151, 152, 156, 163, 180, 232, 259, 276, 281, 286, 300-302, 312, 315, 326, 330-332, 335, 337, 357
completion .. 15-17, 58, 63, 66, 70, 90, 95, 97, 100, 115, 117, 131-133, 135, 138, 144, 157, 160, 161,

165, 166, 177, 196, 203, 258, 266, 268, 280, 296, 306, 309, 313, 326, 334, 337, 352
densities .. 41, 66, 86, 87, 105, 120, 148, 150, 180, 358
eros ... 33, 63, 64, 68, 94, 160, 308, 309, 324
focus . 3, 6, 8-11, 13, 14, 22, 31, 33, 52-55, 59, 61, 63, 64, 67, 70, 75, 82-85, 104, 106, 114, 124, 126-129, 132, 134, 135, 138, 139, 141, 142, 146, 150, 159, 161, 162, 170, 175, 176, 179, 181, 182, 185, 188, 197, 202, 205, 209, 212-214, 219, 221, 236, 243, 247, 250, 262, 272, 284, 285, 293, 296, 299, 300, 304-306, 308, 311, 315, 316, 322, 325, 331, 333, 334, 337, 339, 346, 358
fundamentalism ... 16, 75, 76, 105
headbanging 113
held energy . 57, 68, 72, 76, 77, 81, 95, 105, 112, 121, 125, 142, 155, 156, 171, 172, 183, 220, 254, 302, 307, 312, 319, 323, 326, 334, 335, 353, 359
held-energy system . 76, 79, 80, 83, 85, 87, 88, 92, 94, 99, 101, 106, 108, 115, 116, 122, 124, 127, 131-133, 135, 144-146, 153, 156, 161, 166, 188, 190, 191, 206, 210, 218, 230, 239, 242, 248, 280, 284, 286, 296, 298, 299, 309, 313, 326, 333, 354, 358
impressionism 135
intention ... 19, 38, 41, 43, 66, 134, 135, 143, 145, 161, 165, 177, 179, 270, 272, 275, 322, 343, 348, 358
meditation 55, 59, 86, 104, 135
meditational 44, 114, 135, 145, 147, 162, 165, 305, 332, 341
movement ... 3, 4, 6, 15-17, 23, 29, 30, 36, 40, 44, 53, 59, 63, 66, 71-73, 75, 77, 81, 83, 84, 87, 90-93, 101, 103-105, 111, 113-116, 119, 120, 122, 124, 126, 127, 132, 133, 138, 141, 143-145, 149-151, 153-155, 158, 162, 165, 166, 175, 181, 194, 210,

217, 225, 227, 229, 231, 232, 248, 260, 264, 270, 277, 280, 285-287, 292, 295, 321, 322, 324, 329, 330, 334, 337, 345, 346, 351, 354, 357-359

narrative . . . x, 6, 12, 16, 19, 23, 29, 49-52, 64, 67, 68, 70, 71, 74-76, 79, 81, 84, 85, 89, 90, 92-94, 98, 104, 107, 109-115, 117, 121, 132, 133, 140, 144, 145, 153-157, 159, 160, 162, 165-167, 177, 192, 200, 206, 214, 217, 218, 221, 227, 251, 253, 277, 278, 280, 283, 287, 293, 295-307, 315, 316, 326, 329, 332, 334, 337, 338, 352, 353, 358

pattern . . 4, 6, 7, 12, 13, 16, 20, 22, 23, 28-32, 39, 41, 49, 56, 58, 62, 64-66, 68-72, 75, 76, 79, 82, 83, 85-89, 91, 92, 100, 101, 104, 106, 111, 112, 115, 122, 123, 125-129, 131-134, 136, 138, 140-144, 147, 150, 152, 155, 156, 158, 159, 161, 162, 166, 167, 170, 175-177, 181, 183, 187, 190, 195, 205, 207, 208, 210, 211, 214-218, 223, 224, 227, 228, 236, 238-241, 243, 244, 249, 255, 258, 263, 264, 272, 274, 278, 279, 292, 296, 298, 299, 301, 305, 307, 312, 313, 316, 319, 326, 333, 334, 336, 337, 353, 359

pointillist 116, 142, 171

pre-windshield . . 78-80, 84, 89, 108, 126, 296, 334, 359

scan . . . 76, 105, 106, 122, 124, 132, 133, 158, 180, 187, 207, 358

superstition . 81, 107, 110, 149

symbolist 135

trust . 26, 54, 55, 62, 63, 65, 70, 76, 81, 99, 100, 103, 112, 146, 159, 185, 203, 210, 214, 292, 299, 305, 306, 309, 320, 322-324, 330, 331, 337, 342, 347, 349, 350, 352, 359

trust and trauma . . 99, 103, 323

will . . . 1, 8, 11, 58, 59, 66, 69, 71, 77, 78, 81, 82, 85, 91, 107, 114, 116-118, 121, 122, 124-127, 131-142, 145, 146, 150, 152, 158-161, 165, 167, 171, 172, 176, 177, 185, 188, 189, 192-195, 210, 212, 213, 216, 217, 232, 237, 238, 241, 251, 264, 271-275, 278, 281, 285, 289, 294, 301, 303, 307, 311, 312, 320, 332, 333, 335, 337, 339, 340, 347

witness . . 10, 11, 17, 22, 43, 47, 59, 67, 68, 72, 85, 86, 90, 94, 103, 105, 113, 117, 119, 122, 132, 142, 144, 146, 150, 156, 165, 208, 228, 232, 275, 305, 319, 321, 337, 339, 344

Yale 28, 36-38, 125